PERFECT

HEALTH

PERFECT
HEALTH

The Complete Mind Body Guide

Revised Edition

DEEPAK CHOPRA, M.D.

 THREE RIVERS PRESS • NEW YORK

Published by Three Rivers Press, New York, New York
Member of the Crown Publishing Group.

Random House, Inc. New York, Toronto, London, Sydney, Auckland
www.randomhouse.com

Three Rivers Press is a registered trademark and the Three Rivers Press colophon is a trademark of Random House, Inc.

Originally published in hardcover by Harmony Books in 1991.

Printed in the United States of America

Design by Susan Maksuta

Library of Congress Cataloging-in-Publication Data
Chopra, Deepak.
    Perfect health, revised : the complete mind body guide
  by Deepak Chopra.—1st ed.
    1. Medicine, Psychosomatic.   2. Mind and body.   I. Title.

  RC49.C46   2000
  615.5'3—dc21

                                                    00-032595

ISBN 0-609-80694-7

10   9   8   7   6   5   4   3

Revised Edition

❖

To Shankara
and the
Shankaracharya Tradition of Masters
for preserving the knowledge of
The Wisdom of Life.

❖

Contents

Acknowledgments   *ix*

Part I:
A Place Called Perfect Health

   Introduction   *3*
     1 **Invitation to a Higher Reality**   *7*
     2 **Discovering Your Body Type**   *31*
        Ayurveda Mind Body Type Test   *38*
        Characteristics of the Body Types   *46*
           Vata   *47*
           Pitta   *50*
           Kapha   *53*
        Understanding a Two-Dosha Type   *57*
        Understanding a Three-Dosha Type   *61*
     3 **The Three Doshas—Makers of Reality**   *63*
        The Subdoshas   *77*
     4 **A Blueprint from Nature**   *87*
        How the Doshas Get Unbalanced   *98*
     5 **Restoring the Balance**   *109*
        The Balanced Life—General Points   *121*

Part II:
The Quantum Mechanical Human Body

     6 **Quantum Medicine for a Quantum Body**   *137*
     7 **Opening the Channels of Healing**   *151*
        Panchakarma   *152*
        Meditation   *157*
        Healing Sounds   *167*
        Marma Therapy   *178*
        Aromatherapy   *187*
        Music Therapy   *191*
     8 **Freedom from Addictions**   *197*

Contents

9 Aging Is a Mistake   *213*
  Rasayanas—Herbs for Longevity   *221*
  Quiz: How Well Am I Aging?   *225*

Part III:
Living in Tune with Nature

  10 The Impulse to Evolve   *235*
  11 Daily Routine—Riding Nature's Waves   *243*
  12 Diet—Eating for Perfect Balance   *257*
  Body-Type Diets   *259*
       Vata-Pacifying Diet   *262*
       Pitta-Pacifying Diet   *270*
       Kapha-Pacifying Diet   *276*
  The Six Tastes   *283*
  Agni—The Digestive Fire   *293*
  A Blissful Diet   *306*
  13 Exercise—The Myth of "No Pain, No Gain"   *317*
  Body-Type Exercise   *320*
  Three-Dosha Exercises   *325*
       Sun Salute   *326*
       Yoga Positions   *339*
       Balanced Breathing (*Pranayama*)   *358*
  14 Seasonal Routine—Balancing the Whole Year   *363*

  Epilogue: **Flowers in a Quantum Field**   *369*
  Appendix A: **Sources for Ayurveda**   *377*
  Appendix B: **Glossary**   *381*
  Bibliography   *383*
  Index   *385*

Acknowledgments

I wish to offer my heartfelt thanks:

To my family, for their deep love and support, which is the basis for everything I do.

To David Simon, my friend and colleague, for his support in the updating of this book and the greater vision we share.

To two superb agents—and valued friends—Lynn Franklin and Muriel Nellis, for their belief in this project.

To Huntley Dent, a close friend whose keen literary judgment helped me bring the original text to completed form.

To my editor, Peter Guzzardi, who insists on perfection and bringing out the best I can offer.

And to the dedicated family of doctors, nurses, teachers, and support staff of the Chopra Center for Well Being who are committed to living the ideals of perfect health every day in their lives.

For more information on programs, products, and services to create perfect health, please visit our Web site at www.mypotential.com.

PART I

A PLACE CALLED PERFECT HEALTH

Introduction

Remarkable transformations have occurred in the world since I wrote the first edition of *Perfect Health* almost a decade ago. Ten years ago the ideas that there was more to health than the absence of disease, that natural approaches could enliven our intrinsic healing system, and that the human body was a network of energy and information rather than a frozen anatomical structure seemed radical. And yet today we see that these concepts have become woven into the very fabric of our modern view of health and sickness, and of life and death. A recent report in the *Journal of the American Medical Association* found that over 40 percent of Americans are now regularly accessing unconventional medical care that goes beyond a materialistic view of the human body. More than two in three medical schools have introduced courses on alternative and complementary medicine to their students. And, recognizing that patients are demanding greater choice and access, increasing numbers of insurance companies and health maintenance organizations are covering the costs of holistic medical care.

The scientific community has shifted from outright rejection and ridicule of alternative healing approaches to serious investigation. If you access the National Library of Medicine's database, you will find over forty thousand articles on alternative and complementary medicine with over sixteen hundred on herbal medicines alone. Meditation, yoga, massage, and nutritional approaches are increasingly embraced as mainstream tools for healing. St. John's wort, ginkgo biloba, and echinacea have become household words, with almost every pharmacy in America carrying its own line of natural medicines. Through the proliferation of journals, books, and the Internet, people have unprecedented access to information on health, and are taking increasing responsibility for their own well-being. Although this may be threatening to the established medical community, I see the trend toward increasing self-awareness and empowerment as a sign of expanding personal and collective health.

At the Chopra Center for Well Being in beautiful La Jolla, California, we have created a healing environment to directly explore the power of Ayurveda and mind body medicine. We have developed courses applying the principles and practices of holistic medicine to the most common health concerns. Our Magical Beginnings program provides information and inspiration for pregnant couples to nurture their unborn children as incubating gods and goddesses in embryo. We have certified birth educators around the world teaching this program, which will help create a new generation of healthy, conscious beings.

Mind body educators on every continent in the world have been trained at the Chopra Center to teach Creating Health, our premier course on mind body medicine and Ayurveda. More than five hundred people have been certified worldwide as instructors in Primordial Sound Meditation, our stress-relieving program that enables people to directly experience their inner field of energy and creativity. Return to Wholeness, our course for people facing cancer, has had a transformational effect on those dealing with this challenging illness. Programs for people with chronic fatigue, women transitioning through menopause, and those struggling to lose weight have helped thousands to realize their intrinsic potential to consciously transform their lives. Over the past decade I have repeatedly seen the profound effect that the approaches described in *Perfect Health* have on people's lives.

It has been very gratifying to witness the changes occurring in world consciousness. We are in the midst of a revolution that will forever change the way we view the world and ourselves. The timeless wisdom tradition of Ayurveda and the most advanced theories of modern physics both point to a deeper reality that encourages us to see the universe as an eternal, infinite field of potentiality that we can access for healing and transformation. This is the core message of *Perfect Health*.

This updated version contains some significant changes. I have introduced new healing techniques that we have found useful with patients at the Chopra Center. Guided visualizations and meditations are presented that can provide the direct experience of more expanded awareness, the key to changing your perception of your body. I offer subtle mind body approaches to consciously connect with your cells, tissues, and organs. Learning to influence so-called "autonomic" functions is important in creating and maintaining perfect health. I have updated the sections on nutrition and herbal medicines, with an emphasis on a wholesome, balanced diet. These days, in the rush to ensure health with nutritional supplements, it is important not to overlook the basic health-promoting value of a balanced nutritional program. The Ayurvedic diet promoted in *Perfect Health* is characterized by its simplicity, elegance, and sumptuousness. I have introduced new, updated references, which draw from the growing body of scientific research on mind body interactions in health and sickness. It is very fulfilling to see objective documentation of health principles and practices that go back thousands of years. Expanded ways to nourish your body through the five senses are explored that use healing sound, touch, sight, taste, and smell to awaken the body's inner pharmacy. Understanding that the environment is our extended body, I have introduced fun exercises to enliven the connection between our inner and outer worlds. Overall, this edition of *Perfect Health* is designed to be practical, accessible, and very user-friendly.

In my continuing exploration of healing, I am totally convinced that true health is much more than the absence of an abnormal laboratory finding; it is even more than optimal mind body integration. Health in its essence is a higher state of consciousness. For thousands of years the great Vedic seers have proclaimed that the purpose of attending to the body is to support the state of being known as enlightenment. In this state our internal reference point shifts from the ego to spirit, and we recognize that the knower, the process of knowing, and that which is known are one and the same. The boundaries of time and space become fluid as we remember ourselves as unbounded beings temporarily masquerading as individuals. This state of wholeness is the basis of all healing. This is the state of perfect health. I am grateful for the opportunity to escort you to this place that is very near to where you currently reside.

CHAPTER 1

INVITATION TO A HIGHER REALITY

There exists in every person a place that is free from disease, that never feels pain, that cannot age or die. When you go to this place, limitations which all of us accept cease to exist. They are not even entertained as a possibility.

This is the place called perfect health.

Visits to this place may be very brief, or they may last for many years. Even the briefest visit, however, instills a profound change. As long as you are there, the assumptions that hold true for ordinary existence are altered, and the possibility of a new existence, higher and more ideal, begins to flower. This book is for people who would like to explore this new existence, bring it into their lives, and make it permanent.

The cause of disease is often extremely complex, but one thing can be said for certain: no one has proved that getting sick is necessary. In fact, quite the opposite is true. Every day we come into contact with millions of viruses, bacteria, allergens, and fungi, and only the tiniest fraction of these encounters ever leads to disease. It is not uncommon for doctors to see patients whose respiratory tracts contain clusters of virulent meningococcus bacteria living there harmlessly. Only on rare occasions do they break out and cause meningitis, a serious and at times fatal infection of the central nervous system. Many of us carry the varicella virus, lying dormant in our nerves since a bout with chicken pox as children, but only rarely, under stress, does it reactivate to cause the painful condition of shingles. What provokes such an attack? No one knows precisely, but it seems to involve a mysterious factor called "host resistance," meaning that we, the host of germs, somehow open or close the window to them. More than 99.99 percent of the time, the window is closed, which implies that each of us is much closer to perfect health than we realize.

The leading cause of death in the United States is heart disease, which in most cases is caused by deposits of plaque blocking the coronary arteries that conduct oxygen to the heart. When cholesterol and other debris begin to obstruct these arteries, oxygen starvation threatens to impair the heart's function. Yet the course of heart disease is highly personal. One person with a single, rather small bit of plaque can be incapacitated by angina, the squeezing chest pain symptomatic of coronary artery disease. A second person with several deposits of plaque large enough to block much of the oxygen flow to the heart might feel nothing. People whose coronary arteries were 85 percent blocked have been known to run marathons, while others have dropped dead of a heart attack with completely clean vessels. In fact, recent studies have found that many younger people who die suddenly of a heart attack have none of the usual risk factors for coronary artery disease. Our physical ability to repel disease is extremely flexible.

In addition to our body's physical immunity, we all have strong emotional resistance to sickness. As one woman, an older patient of mine, put it, "I've read enough psychology to know that a well-adjusted adult is supposed to become reconciled to getting sick, growing old, and eventually dying. At some level I have understood that, but emotionally and instinctively, I don't believe it at all. Getting sick and deteriorating physically seem like a ghastly mistake, and I've always hoped someone would come along to correct it."

This woman is nearly 80 now, and her physical and mental condition is excellent. When asked what lies ahead, she said, "You may think this is crazy, but my attitude is that I'm not going to get old, and I'm not going to die." Is that so unreasonable? People who consider themselves "too busy to get sick" are known to have above-average health, while those who worry excessively about disease fall prey to it more often. Another man told us that the idea of perfect health appealed to him because it was a creative solution—perhaps the only solution—to the overwhelming problems currently facing medicine. A highly successful electronics executive, this man compared perfect health to the kind of "breakthrough thinking" that transforms corporations.

Breakthrough thinking is a unique form of problem solving: it involves making a situation better by first raising your expectations much higher than anyone believes possible and then looking for ways to make your vision come true. "If people continue to think and act in the same familiar ways," this man commented, "they may accomplish five to ten percent improvements by working harder. However, to get improvements of two to ten times, targets must be set high enough that people say, 'Well, if you want *that much* improvement, we'll have to do this an entirely different way.'"

Breakthrough thinking has been applied among advanced software companies in Silicon Valley. For example, if the current version of software took two years to develop, the next generation may be scheduled to take only one. If defects in manufacturing have been cut down to 5 percent, then "zero defects" becomes the rule for the future. That is exactly how perfect health works—it sets zero defects as the goal and then explores how the goal can be met. In the high-tech industry, it may cost eight to ten times more to repair a defect than to make it defect-free in the first place. For that reason, imposing "quality at the source" (i.e., doing things right the first time) makes better business sense than going for engineering that is merely good enough.

The same is true in medicine, where prevention is much cheaper than treatment, both in human and economic terms. A recent poll showed that Americans fear catastrophic illness more than anything else. The reason has less to do with pain and suffering than the crushing expense of a long hospital stay and the devastating costs of long-term care. For many people even death is not as frightening as leaving one's family destitute. Clearly, we need a medical approach that believes in "quality at the source" and can promote it in individuals.

PROMISE OF A NEW MEDICINE—AYURVEDA

The first secret you should know about perfect health is that you have to choose it. You can only be as healthy as you think it is possible to be. Perfect health is no mere 5 or 10 percent improvement over good health. It involves a total shift in perspective that makes disease and infirm old age unacceptable.

Can we really believe in "zero defects" for something as complex as the human body? According to the National Institute on Aging, no diet, exercise, vitamin, drug, or lifestyle change has proved itself capable of reliably extending life. Averting the degenerative disorders that afflict the elderly—heart disease, stroke, cancer, arteriosclerosis, arthritis, diabetes, osteoporosis, and so on—is more feasible than ever before but still unlikely. Although in public medical researchers speak optimistically of major breakthroughs in curing cancer and the other major intractable illnesses, they are much more pessimistic among themselves. The best that they hope for is creeping gradualism—taking one tiny step at a time toward a solution. (Lowering cholesterol levels will, statistically, reduce heart attacks in a large group of people, for instance, but it does not guarantee that any single person will be spared.)

To make health twice or ten times better, you need a new kind of knowledge, based on a deeper concept of life. This book presents a unique source of such knowledge, a system of preventive medicine and health care called Ayurveda. Dating back in India more than 5,000 years, Ayurveda comes from two Sanskrit root words, *Ayus*, or "life," and *Veda*, meaning "knowledge" or "science." Therefore, Ayurveda is usually translated as "the science of life." An alternate and more precise reading would be "the knowledge of life span."

The purpose of Ayurveda is to tell us how our lives can be influenced, shaped, extended, and ultimately controlled without interference from sickness or old age. The guiding principle of Ayurveda is that the mind exerts the deepest influence on the body, and freedom from sickness depends upon contacting our own awareness, bringing it into balance, and then extending that balance to the body. This state of balanced awareness, more than any kind of physical immunity, creates a higher state of health.

Ayurveda embodies the collected wisdom of sages who began their tradition many centuries before the construction of the Pyramids and carried it forward generation after generation. At the Chopra Center for Well Being we have developed a modernized system of Ayurveda that integrates the perennial truths of this ancient healing approach with the most advanced insights of modern science.

Over the past fifteen years my colleagues and I have treated more than ten thousand patients and trained nearly three thousand other health care providers in Ayurvedic theory and practice. In adopting Ayurveda, we have not abandoned our conventional training but extended it. Blending Ayurveda and Western medicine brings together ancient wisdom and modern science and the two have proved completely compatible. The doctors at the Chopra Center still take medical histories and work up physicals on their patients, relying on objective tests to tell them when a person is sick. In addition, however, we guide our patients to look inward, to find that all-important balanced awareness inside themselves.

THE QUANTUM MECHANICAL HUMAN BODY

To comprehend how this is possible, we have to delve deeper into the body itself. In Ayurveda, the physical body is the gateway to what I call the "quantum mechanical human body." Physics informs us that the basic fabric of nature lies at the quantum level, far beyond atoms and molecules. A quantum, defined as the basic unit of matter or energy, is from 10,000,000 to 100,000,000 times smaller than the smallest atom. At this level, matter and energy become interchangeable. All quanta are made of invisible vibrations—ghosts of energy—waiting to take physical form. Ayurveda says that the same is true of the human body—it first takes form as intense but invisible vibrations, called quantum fluctuations, before it proceeds to coalesce into impulses of energy and particles of matter.

The quantum mechanical body is the underlying basis for everything we are: thoughts, emotions, proteins, cells, organs—any visible or invisible part of ourselves. At the quantum level, your body is sending out all kinds of invisible signals, waiting for you to pick them up. You have a quantum pulse underlying your physical one, and a quantum heart beating it out. In fact, Ayurveda holds that all the organs and processes in your body have a quantum equivalent.

The quantum mechanical body would do us very little good if we could not detect it. Fortunately, human awareness is capable of sensing these faint vibrations, thanks to the incredible sensitivity of our nervous system. A single photon of light falling upon the retina of the eye makes far less impact than a single speck of dust falling on a football field. Yet the specialized nerve endings of the retina, the rods and cones, can actually detect a single photon, send a message to the brain, and cause you to see its light. Rods and cones are like giant radio telescopes, huge structures that can still gather signals on the very threshold of physical existence, and then amplify them in such a way that our senses can deal with them directly.

By treating the underlying quantum mechanical body itself, Ayurveda can bring about changes far beyond the reach of conventional medicine, confined as it is to the level of gross physiology. This is because the power available at the quantum level is infinitely greater than that found at grosser levels. The explosion of an atom bomb, which is a gigantic quantum event, is but one instance. A more constructive example is the laser, which takes the same light that is emitted by a flashlight, and by organizing it into coherent quantum vibrations boosts its power enough to cut through steel.

What is at work here is the quantum principle, which reveals that the subtlest levels of nature hold the greatest potential energy. The black emptiness of intergalactic space, although a mere vacuum, contains almost inconceivable amounts of hidden energy, enough in every cubic inch to power a star. Only when it makes the quantum leap does this "virtual energy," as it is called, explode into heat, light, and other forms of visible radiation.

We all know that burning a piece of wood releases much less energy than splitting its atoms through a nuclear reaction. But we have ignored the creative side of the same equation—*making* something new at the quantum level would be just as powerful as destroying it. Only nature creates rocks, trees, stars, and galaxies, but we are busily engaged every day in making something arguably far more complex and precious than a star—a human body. Whether we realize it or not, all of us are responsible for creating the body we live in. Headlines were made several years ago when a San Francisco cardiologist, Dr. Dean Ornish, proved that forty advanced heart patients could actually shrink the fatty plaque deposits that were progressively blocking their coronary arteries. As the arteries of these patients began to open, fresh oxygen started reaching their hearts, thus relieving their frightening chest pains and reducing their risk of having fatal coronaries.

Rather than relying on conventional drugs or surgery to unblock their arteries, Dr. Ornish's group used simple yoga exercises, meditation, and a strict vegetarian diet. Recently, Dr. Ornish confirmed that these basic health-promoting lifestyle changes provide long-term benefits in reducing heart disease. Why have these findings been considered so remarkable? Because mainstream medicine had never before acknowledged that heart disease can be reversed once it has started. Medicine's official position is that a sick artery follows its own course of development: No matter what you believe, think, eat, or do, such arteries relentlessly pursue their grim fate, degenerating a little more every day, eventually becoming blocked and strangulating the heart muscle.

Yet, at the quantum level, *no* part of the body lives apart from the rest. There are no wires holding together the molecules of your arteries, just as there are no visible connections binding together the stars in a galaxy. Yet arteries and galaxies are both securely held together, in a seamless, perfect design. The invisible bonds that you cannot examine under a microscope are quantum in nature; without this "hidden physiology," your visible physiology could not exist. It would never have been more than a random collection of molecules.

Ayurveda would say that Ornish's breakthrough for heart disease holds true for any disorder, once you know how to make use of the quantum mechanical body. A deposit of cholesterol-filled plaque looks solid, like rust lining an old pipe, but plaque is alive and changing, just like the rest of the body. New fat molecules drift in and out of it, new capillaries develop to bring in oxygen and food. The real news from Ornish's study is that what we build in our bodies we can also unbuild. A man who dies of a heart attack at age 50 has had innumerable chances to build new arteries. A 70-year-old woman who develops osteoporosis in her spine has had innumerable chances to make a healthy spine. (We cannot really count the chances, since the process of change is constant; however, you could possibly heal a damaged artery or a defective bone in a matter of a few weeks or months.) We are all building new bodies all the time. Why not build a healthy artery, a healthy spine, a complete and healthy person?

In India's ancient Vedic tradition, the most basic force underlying all of nature is intelligence. The universe, after all, is not "energy soup"; it is not mere chaos. The incredibly exact fit of things in our world—above all, the astonishing existence of DNA—argues for an infinite amount of intelligence in nature. As one astrophysicist put it, the likelihood that life was created randomly is about the same as the likelihood that a hurricane could blow through a junkyard and create a Boeing 707.

One of the most crucial changes in contemporary science is the sudden arrival on the scene of models that take intelligence into account as a vital force in the universe. (In physics, for example, there is the so-called anthropic principle, which proposes that the whole of creation since the Big Bang was designed expressly to lead to the existence of man.)

Why is this relevant to us? Because Ayurveda, seen in its larger context, is nothing less than a technology for contacting the quantum level inside ourselves. To get there you need special techniques, which we will cover in detail, that allow you to peel away the mask of the physical body; in addition, you have to transcend, or go beyond, the constant activity that fills the mind, like the noise of a radio that cannot be turned off. Beyond that distraction lies a silent region that appears as empty as the quantum field between the stars. Yet, like that quantum field, our inner silence holds rich promise.

The silence inside us is the key to the quantum mechanical body. It is not a chaotic but an organized silence. It has shape and design, purpose and processes, just like the physical body. Instead of seeing your body as a collection of cells, tissues, and organs, you can use the quantum perspective to see it as a silent flow of intelligence, a constant bubbling up of impulses that create, control, and become your physical body. The secret of life at this level is that *anything in your body* can be changed with the flick of an intention.

You may find this hard to believe, so let me offer the example of Timmy, a perfectly ordinary-seeming 6-year-old who suffers from one of the saddest and strangest of psychiatric syndromes—multiple personality disorder. Timmy has more than a dozen separate personalities, each with its own emotional patterns, vocal inflections, likes and dislikes. Yet people with multiple personalities are not just psychological cases; as they drop one personality and put on another, remarkable changes can occur in their bodies.

One personality might have diabetes, for example, and the person will be insulin-deficient as long as that personality is in force. Yet the other personalities may be completely free of diabetes, testing normally for insulin levels. Likewise, one personality may have high blood pressure while the others do not; even warts, sores, and other skin blemishes have been seen to appear and disappear with the changing of personalities. The literature on multiple personalities includes patients who can instantly alter their pattern of brain waves on an EEG or transform the color of their eyes from blue to brown. One woman had three separate menstrual periods each month, corresponding to her three separate personalities.

Timmy is particularly amazing because one of his personalities, and only one, is allergic to orange juice and breaks out in hives if he drinks it. Health writer Daniel Goleman reported in the *New York Times,* "The hives will occur even if Timmy drinks orange juice and another personality appears while the juice is still being digested. What is more, if Timmy comes back while the allergic reaction is present, the itching of the hives will cease immediately, and the water-filled blisters will begin to subside."

This is a perfect example of how signals from the quantum mechanical body can cause instantaneous changes in the physical body. What is remarkable here is that allergies are not known to come and go at the whim of the mind. How could they? The white cells of the immune system, coated with antibodies that cause the allergic reaction, wait passively for the contact of an antigen. When contact occurs, a series of chemical reactions is triggered automatically.

Yet, in Timmy's case, it appears that as the molecules of orange juice approach his white cells, a *decision* is made whether to react or not. This implies that the cell itself is intelligent. Moreover, its intelligence is contained at a level deeper than its molecules, for the antibody and the orange juice meet end to end with very ordinary atoms of carbon, hydrogen, and oxygen.

To say that molecules can make decisions defies current physical science—it is as if sugar sometimes feels like being sweet and sometimes not. But it is not only the remarkable intensity of Timmy's case that stuns us. Once we absorb the fact that he is choosing to be allergic—for how else could he turn his hives off and on?—then we confront the possibility that we are choosing our own diseases, too. We are not aware of this choice, because it takes place at a level below our everyday thoughts. But if we have such ability, we should be able to control it.

THE BODY IS A RIVER

We all tend to see our bodies as "frozen sculptures"—solid, fixed, material objects—when in truth they are more like rivers, constantly changing, flowing patterns of intelligence. The Greek philosopher Heraclitus declared, "You cannot step into the same river twice, for fresh waters are ever flowing in." The same is true of the body. If you "pinch an inch" around your waist, the fat you are squeezing between your fingers is not the same as it was last month. Your adipose tissues (fat cells) fill up with fat and empty out constantly, so that all of it is exchanged every three weeks. You acquire a new stomach lining every five days (the innermost layer of stomach cells is exchanged in a matter of minutes as you digest food). Your skin is new every five weeks. Your skeleton, seemingly so solid and rigid, is entirely new every three months. In all, the flow of oxygen, carbon, hydrogen, and nitrogen is so rapid that you could be renewed in a matter of weeks; it is only the heavier atoms of iron, magnesium, copper, and so on that slow down the process. You appear to be the same outwardly, yet you are like a building whose bricks are constantly being replaced by new ones. Every year, fully 98 percent of the total number of atoms in your body are replaced—this has been confirmed by radioisotope studies at the Oak Ridge laboratories in California. This constant stream of change is controlled at the quantum level of the mind body system, and yet medicine has not taken advantage of this fact—it is still waiting to take the quantum leap.

To change the printout of the body, you must learn to rewrite the software of the mind. In the following chapters, I would like to lead you on a journey of self-exploration. I will show you how Ayurveda can put you in better control of your health from this quantum level that is the next frontier of medicine. The approach is divided into three parts, corresponding to the three divisions of this book.

PART I: A PLACE CALLED PERFECT HEALTH

First we discuss the possibility of perfect health, then on to practical matters. Ayurveda teaches that every person has been given a unique blueprint by nature; this is called his *prakruti*, or body type. By taking the simple test in chapter 2, you will discover which of the ten basic body types applies to you. This is the most important step toward reaching a higher state of health, because your prakruti tells you how nature intends you to live. According to Ayurveda, your body knows what is good and bad for it; nature has built the correct instincts into you from birth. Once you begin to notice and obey these innate tendencies, you will find that your physiology is capable of achieving balance on its own, with minimal effort on your part.

As we go on to explore, extremely small imbalances in your system sow the seeds of future illness, while preserving balance can ensure an ideal state of health. The strong and weak points of each body type are laid out, enabling you to choose your own specific approach to disease prevention. The sickness you should seek to avoid is the one that you are most prone to, and that is indicated by your prakruti.

PART II: THE QUANTUM MECHANICAL HUMAN BODY

In this section we delve deeper into the quantum level inside ourselves, exploring how the mind directs the body toward sickness and health. Thousands of years before modern medicine discovered the mind body connection, the sages of Ayurveda had mastered it—they developed an "inner technology" that operates from the most profound levels of our awareness. The secret of perfect health lies with the practice of these techniques. We discuss the role of meditation in removing the obstacles to health; we explore how the quantum mechanical human body can be exploited to change the physical body far more powerfully than can any drug, diet, or exercise.

In this section we range widely through many subjects, from addictions to cancer to removal of physical and mental toxins—all the areas of medicine that are treated at the Chopra Center for Well Being. By seeing yourself through the eyes of an Ayurvedic doctor and reading case studies of people who have gone through our programs, you will better understand why "quantum healing" represents a major advance in our approach to mind and body.

PART III: LIVING IN TUNE WITH NATURE

After presenting the grand design of Ayurveda, I end with the practical advice I have gleaned over the past fifteen years. The ideal of perfect health depends upon perfect balance. Everything you eat, say, think, do, see, and feel affects your overall state of balance. It would seem impossible to control all these different influences at once. Yet, by following specific body-type diets, exercises, and daily and seasonal routines, you can correct the vast majority of imbalances now present in your physiology and prevent those that might lie in the future.

THE REENCHANTMENT OF NATURE

It is fascinating to see how perfect health dovetails into a broader intellectual movement that is rocking the foundations of science. Ilya Prigogine, Nobel Prize winner in chemistry in 1977 and a pioneer in this movement, calls it "the reenchantment of nature"—the realization that nature is not a machine but a wondrous environment whose hidden possibilities are barely guessed at today. Nature is like a radio band with infinite stations; the reality you are now experiencing is only one station on the band, completely convincing as long as you stay tuned to it, but masking the other choices that lie on either side.

At the turn of the century, psychologist William James hinted at the mechanism that allows us to turn the dial: "One of the greatest discoveries of my generation," he wrote, "was that human beings can alter their lives by altering their attitudes of mind." This was a very farseeing remark, aimed more at the future than at James's time. In his day it was undisputed that nature unfolded mechanically, the result of inflexible laws operating without regard for human beings. Now it appears that human beings actually may count for a lot—perhaps nature is giving us only the reality we expect and believe in.

Certainly we have spent many centuries believing in disease and dying. This says much more about our relation to life than it does about life itself. Life is immensely flexible, and the forces that cause it to endure are at least as strong as those that cause it to decay. If you plant a bristlecone pine on a downtown lot in a polluted city, it may live for fifty years; planted in the country, its life span may increase to two or three hundred years; on the windswept ridges of the Rocky Mountains, it might survive more than two thousand years. Which life span is its natural one? It depends entirely on the situation. Some forces are always working to preserve the bristlecone's life, others to oppose it. In that dynamic balance lies the tree's destiny. Both a relatively short life and an immensely long one are natural, depending on the environment.

A laboratory mouse will typically live fewer than two years raised in a cage on a normal diet. If you lower its body temperature and feed it a minimal amount of calories (while still preserving the vitamins, minerals, protein, and so on that it needs), the mouse's life span can be extended twice or even three times as long. On the other hand, if you expose the same mouse to abnormal stress, such as tossing it every day in front of a cat that is kept just out of reach, the mouse will very likely die in a matter of weeks. In every case, the mouse's internal organs will have aged to the same degree—the worn-out heart, liver, and kidneys will be uniformly "old," even though the oldest mouse lived perhaps fifty times longer than the youngest.

As the balance of forces change, life changes. In the case of human beings, environment can be chosen and controlled, which gives our own life spans enormous flexibility. When we speak of perfect health, we are proposing that the dynamic balance of life can be tipped to our advantage. No one has lived forever, but you can add 50 years to an average, modern life span of 70 years and reach the longest life span on record (121 years, credited to an offshore Japanese islander). In the Roman Empire, adult life expectancy was 28 years; by the year 2020 it may rise to 90 years for a healthy American, male or female. That represents a great deal of flexibility.

If you look at the smallest unit of life—the cell—the discrepancy between a long and a short life is even more pronounced. Fetch a pail of water from the edge of a pond. When you put a drop under a microscope, it will be teeming with one-celled plants and animals—paramecia, amoebae, algae, and so on. Each amoeba may have a life span of only two or three weeks. But because amoebae multiply by division, the genetic material inside each amoeba is as old as the mother cell it came from, which makes it four weeks old instead of two. The mother cell descended from its own mother, so you would have to say that part of the amoeba you are looking at is three times as old as you thought, part of it four times as old, until you come to the conclusion that, in part, this single amoeba from your local pond is as old as all the amoebae that have ever lived, perhaps a billion years.

The actual atoms and molecules inside the amoeba have not inhabited it for that long. They come and go constantly, in a swirl of oxygen, hydrogen, carbon, and nitrogen. Nevertheless, the amoeba retains its shape and identity generation after generation. Some living force holds it together, and as long as the amoeba's DNA is not destroyed, this cell will house its portion of life forever.

Your body, composed of between 50 and 100 trillion cells, is inconceivably more complex than an amoeba, but you are housing life that is just as old and just as young at the same time. To speak accurately about the human life span, you must refer to the many life spans represented inside one body.

A typical cell in the lining of your stomach lives only a few days and a typical skin cell only two weeks; a red blood cell lives longer—two or three months. Very long-lived cells can be found in the liver, where they take several years to replace themselves; heart and brain cells apparently last a lifetime without reproducing.

The amazing thing is that the exact same DNA controls all these life spans, from the very shortest to the very longest. Skin cells and brain cells are genetically identical; they are descended from the moment of conception, when half of your father's DNA fused with half of your mother's to form the unique strand of DNA that became you. Through a process we are just beginning to understand, your DNA was able to create all kinds of specialized cells—brain, skin, heart, liver, and so on—each with its own allotted life span. You cannot tell which life will be long or short just by looking at the cell: the neurons in your brain, many of which last a lifetime, are all but identical to the olfactory cells in your nose, which give you your sense of smell, yet olfactory cells are replaced every four weeks.

Like the amoeba, each human cell is made of atoms that literally fly through it—it takes only a few thousandths of a second to exchange oxygen and carbon dioxide in your lungs; sodium and potassium ions are pumped in and out of brain cells three hundred times per second. Your heart muscle extracts oxygen out of the blood's hemoglobin so quickly that in a few seconds the blood feeding the heart via the coronary arteries, which is bright red in color, exits almost black.

But this endless swirl of activity doesn't dissolve your shape or identity, any more than it does the amoeba's. Your DNA has been distinctly humanlike for several million years; the primeval DNA it is descended from is as old as life itself, dating back almost 2 billion years. You are exceedingly permanent at the genetic level, although the material of your body comes and goes.

LIFE FREE FROM IMPERFECTIONS

If life can be so flexible and dynamic, the wonder is that we do not last longer. And we would, if we knew how to handle the balance of forces that are at work in and around us. The ancient sages of Ayurveda were bold enough to ask the ultimate question: Must we become sick and grow old at all? Their answer was no. If the forces inside us are kept in harmony and in balance with the surrounding environment, we can be immune to illness. Perfect balance makes perfect health possible.

In Ayurveda we rely on the basic principle that any disorder can be prevented as long as balance is maintained, not just in the body, but in the mind and spirit as well. The Ayurvedic sages teach that there is an impulse in all of us to grow and progress. This impulse governs our overall balance automatically; it can be seen at work in every cell, but particularly in the brain, which simultaneously balances body temperature, metabolic rate, growth, hunger and thirst, sleep, blood chemistry, respiration, and numerous other functions. Their coordination must be incredibly precise for health to be maintained (the hypothalamus, a tiny region of the forebrain no bigger than a fingertip, coordinates dozens of the body's automatic functions, earning it the nickname "the brain's brain").

But the real source of balance goes deeper still, to the quantum level. Here our basic impulse to grow and progress can be tapped through special techniques that we will explore. This is a vital and yet largely unknown area to most people, which is why they frequently find themselves helpless in the face of illness and aging. When the forces acting against life gain the upper hand, the body has no choice but to deteriorate over time.

On the other hand, if we learn to live in balance from the deepest level, our inner growth has no foreseeable limits. Dozens of books expound the value of inner growth, but they miss the key ingredient that Ayurveda emphasizes: Growth is automatic; it is in nature's plan, built into our very cells. It is only a question of following the silent river of intelligence to its source. That is the final secret of perfect health. If we could allow the mind to expand and to explore higher realities, the body would follow. Wouldn't that be enough to save it from disease and old age?

We can only speculate how far evolution will take us, but there are dramatic instances where the mind refused to believe in disease and the body suddenly followed. Not long ago I saw a Swiss patient named Andreas Schmitt who had been diagnosed with a fatal cancer. A year and a half earlier he noticed a sore spot on his back that bothered him whenever he leaned back in his chair.

Exploring with his fingers, he detected a swollen area about the size of a dime. His wife said it looked like an enlarged dark mole; angling with his wife's hand mirror, Andreas caught a glimpse of a purplish-brown growth located squarely between his shoulder blades.

Events moved quickly and grimly after that. An oncologist in Geneva took a biopsy, which revealed the presence of melanoma, the most virulent and fastest-spreading form of skin cancer. Within a day Andreas was operated on. The surgeons removed the growth and explored the lymph nodes under the right armpit. Fourteen suspected nodes were removed; four of them turned out to have melanoma cells inside. Now that the original melanoma was gone, the next step was to radiate the sites on his back and shoulder to catch any stray cancer cells that might remain. Andreas, a well-educated man in his early fifties, refused the radiation.

"My logic," he told me later, "was just to wait and see. The tumor was gone; I had suffered considerable trauma from the surgery, and inside I wasn't sure that I felt strong enough to submit to more treatments. If I had time to recover at home and build up my confidence, wouldn't I be better off?"

This decision disturbed his oncologist, who said that if Andreas discontinued treatment, his melanoma would almost surely be back in six months.

"And with radiation it won't?" Andreas asked.

"The chances will be smaller," his doctor said.

"And how much longer can I expect to live after that?" Andreas asked.

His doctor was forced into an uneasy guess. Untreated, metastatic melanoma patients may live only a few months; treated to the maximum, their life expectancy stretches out, sometimes by a few years, sometimes not. After five years, the number of long-term survivors is under 10 percent. Within ten years, virtually no one is left alive.

"So if I am not going to survive in the long run," Andreas said, "why go through the agony just to please some doctor?"

His life moved ahead for the next six months, until a swollen lymph node appeared, this time under his left armpit. Tests revealed it to be the return of melanoma, as predicted. At this point, no realistic medical hope remained. When Andreas came to America for help, I first introduced him to the concept of the quantum mechanical body. "Before a cancer can exist physically, it must be triggered at a deeper level. Rather than talking about the breakdown of DNA's self-repair mechanism or the action of carcinogens, Ayurveda says that illness results from distortions in the patterns of quantum vibrations that hold the body intact.

"You can learn to take your awareness to that subtle level of yourself—in fact, what we call thoughts and emotions are just expressions of these quantum fluctuations. Awareness has the capacity to heal, and it seems to be instrumental in causing sudden cures even in the most advanced cases of incurable disease."

All so-called incurable illnesses have instances of unexplained cures. One of the peculiarities of melanoma is that it is more subject to self-cure than many much less deadly forms of cancer. These "spontaneous remissions" are comparatively rare, happening far less than 1 percent of the time, but they can apparently result in full, lasting recoveries.

"If one person has cured himself of melanoma," I pointed out, "then we know it is possible. What triggers it? Some new discovery that you have to make inside yourself. Right now, you stand as good a chance of making this discovery as anyone."

Despite the odds against him, Andreas took this advice seriously. He learned several Ayurvedic approaches to activate his healing forces and underwent purification treatments to remove impurities from his body (this approach is explained in chapters 6 and 7). Our focus was improving his immediate quality of life. He returned to Switzerland and four months later he reported jubilantly that his swollen lymph node had subsided. X rays and blood tests revealed no trace of melanoma in his body. Although Swiss oncologists had not expected him to live more than three months after the recurrence of his cancer, Andreas is leading a normal life several years later.

The most striking aspect of this case is that the patient's mind invited his body to accept a new reality, and it did, oblivious of the fact that what was happening was "impossible." How can we explain such extraordinary events? A study of four hundred cancer cases that went into spontaneous remission revealed cures that had little in common. Some people drank grape juice or swallowed massive doses of vitamin C; others prayed, took herbal remedies, or simply cheered themselves on. These very diverse patients did have one thing in common, though. At a certain point in their disease, they suddenly knew, with complete certainty, that they were going to get better, as if the disease were merely a mirage, and the patient suddenly passed beyond it into a space where fear and despair and all sickness were nonexistent.

They entered the place called perfect health.

CHAPTER 2

DISCOVERING YOUR BODY TYPE

It's a clear October day in downtown Boston (or New York, or Chicago), and the lunch crowd is on its way back to work. Some people are dressed in hats, scarves, and gloves, anticipating winter; others, wearing short-sleeved shirts, seem to think it's still summer. Running bare-chested in shorts, a jogger jumps the green light at the curb, heading for the park. He stands out in vivid contrast to an older woman waiting for her bus bundled in a full-length coat with a fur collar. At a casual glance, you would think these people lived in different climates. Actually, they are expressing the differences nature has created inside themselves.

Despite the fact that many people had a typical lunch of sandwich, French fries, and coffee, the food is sitting heavily in some stomachs, tossing nervously in others, and passing unnoticed in most of the rest. In some bodies, hearts are beating faster because the sidewalk feels too crowded; others are pouring out excess gastric acid or experiencing a rise in blood pressure. It takes all types to make a world—but has medicine really noticed what types there are?

In conventional medicine we pay much more attention to differences among diseases than among people. If a patient complains of a twinge of arthritis in his hands, a physician realizes that this common complaint may be linked to over a hundred diseases, all of which lead to sore, stiff, inflamed, painful joints. It is known that some people inherit the tendency to become arthritic, but a bewildering number of things also seem to contribute—hormonal changes, physical and mental stress, diet, lack of exercise, and so on.

Ayurveda points out that diseases differ mainly because people are so different. Although biology does acknowledge that all of us were born with "biochemical individuality," this has few practical implications in the doctor's office. Biochemical individuality means that no one is average. At any given moment, your cells and tissues do not contain an average level of oxygen, carbon dioxide, iron, insulin, or vitamin C. Instead, they contain a precise amount unique to that moment, to the physical condition of your body, and to the state of your thoughts and emotions. Your body is a three-dimensional composite of millions of tiny differences, and by learning about them you can make dramatic improvements in your health. At this level, perfect health is a very specific biological phenomenon.

THE FIRST STEP—KNOWING YOUR BODY TYPE

Everywhere you look, your body is doing something unique with every molecule of air, water, and food you take in, guided by its innate tendencies. You have the choice to follow these tendencies or modify them, but to recklessly oppose them is unnatural. In Ayurveda, living in tune with nature—easily, comfortably, and without strain—means respecting your uniqueness.

The first question an Ayurvedic doctor asks is not, "What disease does my patient have?" but, "Who is my patient?" By "who" he does not mean your name but how you are constituted. He looks for the telltale traits that disclose your body type, also known as your *prakruti*. This Sanskrit term means "nature"—it is your basic nature he wants to uncover before he turns to your complaints and symptoms.

The Ayurvedic body type is like a blueprint outlining the innate tendencies that have been built into your system. A glass of whole milk contains 120 calories, no matter who drinks it, but one person uses those calories mainly to store fat, while another converts most of it into energy. A child's body extracts lots of calcium to build new bone tissue, while an older person passes the same calcium out through his kidneys (and may convert it into a painful kidney stone if his body can no longer deal efficiently with calcium).

By knowing your body type, an Ayurvedic doctor can tell which diet, physical activities, and medical therapies should help you and which might do no good or even cause harm. A pizza with extra cheese can be potentially lethal to someone with advanced artery disease, for example—the fat ingested could be the last straw that ruptures one of the deposits of fatty plaque blocking a blood vessel to the heart. Massive heart attacks have resulted from the tiniest of these ruptures. Yet the same pizza would be relatively harmless to the rest of us; high fat is even desirable for those who cannot gain weight on normal diets. Knowing who you are—your prakruti—is an invaluable clue to what you should eat.

There are three important reasons why knowing your body type is the first step toward perfect health:

1. *The seeds of disease are sown early.* It would be hard to find a heart patient in his forties who had not shown some suspicious signs in his twenties. A pathologist examining the arteries of a deceased 20-year-old can see premature streaks of fat

that are liable to create a future heart attack. Even 10-year-olds will already be prone either to allergies or to chronic over-weight, high cholesterol, or peptic ulcers. But at this age, when incipient disease is easiest to treat and prevent, symptoms are often difficult to read. By understanding body types and their specific strengths and weaknesses, you can begin to take preventive steps when they do the most good, long before overt illness appears.

2. *Body types make prevention more specific.* Nobody is prone to every disease, yet most of us try to prevent as many as we can—cancer, heart attacks, osteoporosis, and so on—moving uncertainly from one medical scare to the next. If you try to prevent every disease without knowing your particular predisposition, you are stabbing in the dark. Why do 60 million American adults go around with untreated high blood pressure? At least part of the reason is that there is not enough personal connection being made between prevention and the individual who needs it. Heart attacks, cancer, and diabetes happen to specific people, one by one. It only makes sense that prevention must proceed on the same basis.

3. *Body types make treatment more accurate once a disease appears.* Generalized treatment—prescribing Valium to everyone who is anxious or antacids to everyone who has an ulcer—is a hit-or-miss affair; it assumes that a given disease is the same in all people. But as we have seen, this is not true. According to Ayurveda, three people may feel anxious at three different levels of stress. Their ulcers may result from three different diets, job pressures, or difficulties at home. In effect, they are suffering from three different diseases, all of which happen to travel under the same name. This is true for people who chain-smoke, compulsively overeat, or suffer from allergies and asthma. In all these cases, the Ayurvedic body type is

remarkably accurate, as you will see, because it can pinpoint what is happening inside each individual.

Finally, knowing your body type is essential to understanding yourself. When you find out what is actually going on inside, you will no longer be bound by society's notions of what you should be doing, saying, thinking, and feeling. One of the delights of learning about Ayurveda is its insight into little things you probably dismiss as idiosyncrasies. On TV everybody is urged to drink a glass of orange juice in the morning, but some people get heartburn or an upset stomach from it. This is not abnormal; it is a sign that they fall into a specific body type for which the acid quality of orange juice is not ideal.

A person whose nerves are jangled by a cup of weak coffee is by nature different from someone who downs three cups of black espresso without feeling a thing. When you react to a cup of coffee, a cold draft, criticism from your boss, a love note, or rainy weather, your body type is sending you a signal. It is a very personal signal that you alone can tune in to. If you start to listen to all these signals that are sent to you day by day, minute by minute, you will notice that they affect your moods, behavior, perceptions, tastes, talents, attraction to other people, and much more.

The phrase "body type" is only a hint at what prakruti means—it is really your world, the personal reality you generate from the creative core inside. More accurately, we might call your prakruti your "psycho-physiological constitutional type," a phrase that includes both mind (psyche) and body (physiology). I am avoiding this phrase for the sake of brevity, but it is worth remembering that your physical body type has a mental aspect as well.

THE BODY'S SWITCHING STATION

Where do body types come from? Everyone has essentially the same kinds of cells and organs, even though genetics may dictate that you were born with blue eyes instead of brown. And despite huge variations from one personality to the next, we also share the same range of emotions. To find the deeper origin of body types, Ayurveda looks at the meeting point between mind and body. Clearly the two do meet. Every time there is an event in the mind, there is a corresponding event in the body. If a child is afraid of the dark, his fear takes physical shape in the form of adrenaline shooting through his bloodstream. Ayurveda says that this interconnectedness is accomplished at a place sandwiched between mind and body, where thought turns into matter; it is occupied by three operating principles called *doshas*.

The doshas are unique and extremely important, because they allow the mind's dialogue with the body. All your hopes, fears, dreams, and wishes, along with the faintest wisps of emotion and desire, have left their marks on your physiology—these mental events constantly shape the body as they "talk" to it. For most of us, the messages are not as life-supporting as they should be. At some point in our adult lives, the marks of stress and age begin to prevail over those of growth and expansion. If your mind is capable of love and creativity while your body wears out year by year, the doshas need attention.

According to Ayurveda, the reason the downward drag of entropy overcomes the upward pull of evolution lies here: Imbalance in the doshas is the first sign that mind and body are not perfectly coordinated. This is why a poet as brilliant as Keats dies at 26 of tuberculosis and a musical genius on the order of Mozart dies of kidney disease when he is only 35.

The mind's genius was not coupled to the body. On the other hand, restoring the doshas opens up the possibility of a mind body system that is always balanced, always healthy, always evolving.

The three doshas are called Vata, Pitta, and Kapha. Although they regulate thousands of separate functions in the mind body system, they have three basic functions:

Vata dosha controls movement.
Pitta dosha controls metabolism.
Kapha dosha controls structure.

Every cell in your body has to contain all three of these principles. To remain alive, your body has to have Vata, or motion, which allows it to breathe, circulate blood, pass food through the digestive tract, and send nerve impulses to and from the brain. It has to have Pitta, or metabolism, which processes food, air, and water throughout the entire system. It has to have Kapha, or structure, to hold the cells together and form muscle, fat, bone, and sinew. Nature needs all three to build a human body.

In the following chapter we will delve deeper into the doshas. First, though, we must determine your body type, which will give you a much more personal interest in the doshas. Just as there are three doshas, there are three basic types of human constitution in the Ayurvedic system, depending upon which of the doshas is dominant. If a doctor examines you and says, "You are a Vata type," he means that Vata characteristics are the most prominent in you; you would be said to have a Vata prakruti.

The importance of knowing that you are a Vata type—or a Pitta or a Kapha—is that it sharply focuses your diet, exercise, daily routine, and other measures for preventing disease. A Vata person lives in a Vata-colored world down to the smallest detail. By eating food that he knows will balance Vata, he can exert a tremendous balancing influence everywhere. This will become obvious to you as soon as you complete the quiz on the following pages. Please remember, however, that all three doshas are present in everyone, and all three need to be kept in balance. The knowledge of body type that you will gain is your key to *total* balance; it provides the all-important ingredient for change—yourself as nature made you.

AYURVEDA MIND BODY TYPE TEST

The following quiz is divided into three sections. For the first 20 questions, which apply to Vata dosha, read each statement and mark, from 1 to 6, how well it applies to you.

> 1 = Doesn't apply to me
> 3 = Applies to me somewhat (or some of the time)
> 6 = Applies to me very much (or nearly all of the time)

At the end of the section, write down your total Vata score. For example, if you mark a 6 for the first question, a 3 for the second, and a 2 for the third, your total up to that point would be 6 + 3 + 2 = 11. Total the entire section in this way, and you arrive at your final score. Proceed to the 20 questions for Pitta and those for Kapha.

When you are finished, you will have three separate scores. Comparing these will determine your body type.

For fairly objective physical traits, your choice will usually be obvious. For mental traits and behavior, which are more subjective, you should answer according to how you have felt and acted most of your life, or at least for the past few years.

SECTION 1—VATA

	Does Not Apply	Sometimes Applies	Applies Most

1. I perform activity very quickly.
   1 • 2 • 3 • 4 • 5 • ⓺ (A)

2. I am not good at memorizing things and then remembering them later.
   1 • 2 • 3 • 4 • ⑤ • 6 (A)

3. I am enthusiastic and vivacious by nature.
   1 • 2 • 3 • ④ • 5 • 6 (A)

4. I have a thin physique—I don't gain weight very easily.
   1 • 2 • 3 • ④ • 5 • 6 (A)

5. I learn new things easily.
   1 • 2 • 3 • 4 • ⑤ • 6 (A)

6. My characteristic gait while walking is light and quick.
   1 • 2 • 3 • ④ • 5 • 6 (A)

7. I tend to have difficulties making decisions.
   ① • 2 • 3 • 4 • 5 • 6 (A)

8. I tend to develop gas or become constipated easily.
   1 • 2 • 3 • 4 • 5 • ⓺ (A)

9. I tend to have cold hands and feet.
   1 • 2 • 3 • ④ • 5 • 6 (A)

10. I become anxious or worried frequently.
    1 • 2 • 3 • ④ • 5 • 6 (A)

11. I don't tolerate cold weather as well as most people.
    1 • ② • 3 • 4 • 5 • 6 (A)

12. I speak quickly and my friends think I am talkative.
    1 • 2 • ③ • 4 • 5 • 6 (A)

13. My moods change easily and I am somewhat emotional by nature.
    1 • 2 • 3 • ④ • 5 • 6 (A)

14. I often have difficulty in falling asleep or having a sound night's sleep.
    1 • ② • 3 • 4 • 5 • 6 (A)

	Does Not Apply	Sometimes Applies	Applies Most

15. My skin tends to be dry, especially in winter.
1 • 2 • 3 • 4 • ⑤ • 6 *(A above 5)*

16. My mind is very active, sometimes restless, but also very imaginative.
1 • 2 • 3 • ④ • 5 • 6 *(A above 5)*

17. My movements are quick and active; my energy tends to come in bursts.
1 • 2 • ③ • 4 • 5 • 6 *(A above 5)*

18. I am easily excitable.
1 • 2 • ③ • 4 • 5 • 6 *(A above 5)*

19. Left on my own, my eating and sleeping habits tend to be irregular.
1 • ② • 3 • 4 • 5 • 6

20. I learn quickly, but I also forget quickly.
1 • 2 • 3 • ④ • 5 • 6 *(A above 2)*

VATA SCORE _____ 71

A 75

SECTION 2—PITTA

	Does Not Apply	Sometimes Applies	Applies Most

1. I consider myself to be very efficient.
1 • 2 • 3 • 4 • ⑤ • 6 *(A above 5)*

2. In my activities, I tend to be extremely precise and orderly.
1 • 2 • 3 • 4 • ⑤ • 6 *(A above 4)*

3. I am strong-minded and have a somewhat forceful manner.
1 • 2 • 3 • ④ • 5 • 6 *(A above 6)*

4. I feel uncomfortable or become easily fatigued in hot weather—more so than most other people.
1 • 2 • 3 • 4 • 5 • ⑥ *(A above 3)*

	Does Not Apply	Sometimes Applies	Applies Most

5. I tend to perspire easily. 1 • 2 • 3 • 4 • ⑤ • 6   (A)

6. Even though I might not always show it, I become irritable or angry quite easily. 1 • 2 • 3 • ④ • 5 • 6   (A)

7. If I skip a meal or a meal is delayed, I become uncomfortable. 1 • 2 • 3 • 4 • ⑤ • 6   (A)

8. One or more of the following characteristics describes my hair:
    early graying or balding
    thin, fine, straight hair
    blond, red, or sandy colored hair 1 • 2 • 3 • ④ • 5 • 6   (H)

9. I have a strong appetite; if I want to, I can eat quite a large quantity. 1 • 2 • 3 • ④ • 5 • 6   (A)

10. Many people consider me stubborn. 1 • 2 • ③ • 4 • 5 • 6   (A)

11. I am very regular in my bowel habits—it would be more common for me to have loose stools than to be constipated. 1 • 2 • 3 • ④ • 5 • 6   (A)

12. I become impatient very easily. 1 • 2 • 3 • ④ • 5 • 6   (A)

13. I tend to be a perfectionist about details. 1 • 2 • 3 • 4 • ⑤ • 6   (A)

14. I get angry quite easily, but then quickly forget about it. 1 • 2 • ③ • 4 • 5 • 6   (A)

15. I am very fond of cold foods like ice cream and also crave ice-cold drinks. 1 • 2 • 3 • ④ • 5 • 6   (A)

16. I am more likely to feel that a room is too hot than too cold. 1 • 2 • 3 • 4 • ⑤ • 6   (A)

	Does Not Apply	Sometimes Applies	Applies Most

17. I don't tolerate foods that are very hot and spicy.　　1 • 2 • 3 • (4) • 5 • 6

18. I am not very tolerant of disagreement.　　1 • 2 • (3) • 4 • 5 • 6

19. I enjoy challenges and when I want something, I am very determined in my efforts to get it.　　1 • 2 • (3) • 4 • 5 • 6

20. I tend to be critical of others and also of myself.　　1 • 2 • 3 • (4) • 5 • 6

PITTA SCORE ___84___　　69

SECTION 3—KAPHA

	Does Not Apply	Sometimes Applies	Applies Most

1. My natural tendency is to do things in a slow and relaxed fashion.　　1 • (2) • 3 • 4 • 5 • 6

2. I gain weight more easily than most people and lose it more slowly.　　1 • 2 • (3) • 4 • 5 • 6

3. I have a placid and calm disposition—I'm not easily ruffled.　　1 • 2 • (3) • 4 • 5 • 6

4. I can skip meals easily without any significant discomfort.　　1 • (2) • 3 • 4 • 5 • 6

5. I have a tendency toward excess mucus, phlegm, chronic congestion, asthma, or sinus problems.　　1 • 2 • 3 • 4 • (5) • 6

	Does Not Apply	Sometimes Applies	Applies Most

6. I must get at least eight hours of sleep in order to be comfortable the next day.

1 • 2 • ③ • 4 • 5 • 6̂

7. I sleep very deeply.

1 • 2 • 3̂ • 4 • ⑤ • 6

8. I am calm by nature and not easily angered.

1̂ • 2 • ③ • 4 • 5 • 6

9. I don't learn as quickly as some people, but I have excellent retention and a long memory.

1 • ②̂ • 3 • 4 • 5 • 6

10. I have a tendency toward becoming plump—I store extra fat easily.

1 • 2 • ③ • 4̂ • 5 • 6

11. Weather that is cool and damp bothers me.

1 • 2 • ③̂ • 4 • 5 • 6

12. My hair is thick, dark, and wavy.

1̂ • 2 • ③ • 4 • 5 • 6

13. I have smooth, soft skin with a somewhat pale complexion.

1̂ • 2 • ③ • 4 • 5 • 6

14. I have a large, solid body build.

1 • 2 • ③ • 4 • 5̂ • 6

15. The following words describe me well: serene, sweet-natured, affectionate, and forgiving.

1 • 2̂ • 3 • ④ • 5 • 6

16. I have slow digestion, which makes me feel heavy after eating.

1 • 2 • ③ • 4̂ • 5 • 6

17. I have very good stamina and physical endurance as well as a steady level of energy.

1 • 2 • ③ • 4 • 5̂ • 6

18. I generally walk with a slow, measured gait.

①̂ • 2 • 3 • 4 • 5 • 6

	Does Not Apply	Sometimes Applies	Applies Most

19. I have a tendency toward oversleeping, grogginess upon awakening, and am generally slow to get going in the morning.

(1) • 2 • 3 • 4 • 5 • 6   [4 above 5]

20. I am a slow eater and am slow and methodical in my actions.

1 • (2) • 3 • 4 • 5 • 6   [4 above 2]

KAPHA SCORE ___53___

FINAL SCORE
Vata ___75___   Pitta ___84___   Kapha ___57___
75   69   60

DETERMINING YOUR BODY TYPE

Although there are only three doshas, Ayurveda combines them in ten possible ways to arrive at ten different body types.

SINGLE-DOSHA TYPES:

Vata

Pitta

Kapha

If one dosha is much higher than the others, you are a single-dosha type. Most indicative is a score where the primary dosha is twice as high as the second (for example, Vata–90, Pitta–45, Kapha–35), but smaller margins also count. A true single-dosha type displays the traits of Vata, Pitta, or Kapha very prominently. Your next highest dosha will still show some influence in your natural tendencies but to a much lesser degree.

TWO-DOSHA TYPES:

> Vata-Pitta or Pitta-Vata
> Pitta-Kapha or Kapha-Pitta
> Kapha-Vata or Vata-Kapha

If no dosha is extremely dominant, you are a two-dosha type. This means that you display qualities of your two leading doshas, either side by side or in alternation. The higher one comes first in your body type, but both count.

Most people are two-dosha types. In some, the first dosha is very strong—they have scores like Vata–70, Pitta–90, Kapha–46, which would qualify as pure Pitta except for the prominence of another dosha, Vata. In other cases, where the difference is smaller, the first dosha still predominates, but the second will be almost equal. Your score might be Vata–85, Pitta–80, Kapha–40, which is a Vata-Pitta type, even though these two doshas are very close.

Finally, some people have scores in which one dosha stands out but the other two are exactly tied (for example, V–69, P–86, K–69). They are still likely to be a two-dosha type, but a written test did not pick up the second dosha—this person is either a Pitta-Vata or a Pitta-Kapha. If your score is like this, pay attention to the first dosha as your dominant one, and with time the second will become clearer.

THREE-DOSHA TYPE: VATA-PITTA-KAPHA

If your three scores are nearly equal (for example, Vata–88, Pitta–75, Kapha–82), you are a three-dosha type. This type is considered rare, however. Check your answers over carefully, or have a friend help you take the test again to verify your responses. Then read over the descriptions of Vata, Pitta, and Kapha in the following pages to see if one or two doshas are prominent in your makeup. If not, we discuss the three-dosha type more fully on page 61.

Vata Creates Confusion. If you find yourself unable to give clear-cut answers on many points, your body type may be obscured by a Vata imbalance. Vata is the "leader of the doshas" and can mimic Pitta and Kapha. You may be thin-framed but also overweight; prone to worry but also irritable; or you may have insomnia for a stretch of time followed by oversleeping. Vata imbalance is likely to cause such change-ableness.

At bottom, body types are generally not ambiguous. As you gain more understanding of the Ayurvedic system, you will be able to see which answers were due to Vata imbalance and which to your true nature. If you remain confused, consultation with an Ayurvedic physician is advised.

CHARACTERISTICS OF THE BODY TYPES

Having determined your body type, you can now learn to interpret it. One important thing to know about the Ayurvedic system is that it is genetic. Body types are inherited. Long before the theory of DNA, the Ayurvedic sages realized that genetic traits come in groups: Oriental skin and hair come with brown eyes, not blue ones; solid musculature comes with heavy bones to support it, not light, thin ones. Mind, body, and behavior are consistently packaged together in subtle ways that are revealed only by knowledge of the doshas.

Your body type is the mold you were cast in, but it does not contain your fate. To be tall or short, indecisive or determined, anxious or calm is to be a type, yet there is abundant room for all the things that a body type does not control—thoughts, emotions, memories, talents, desires, and so forth. *Knowledge of your body type enables you to evolve to a more ideal state of health.* Unlike Western medicine, which aims at only physical or mental health, Ayurveda wants to lift every aspect of life to a higher level—personal relationships, work satisfaction, spiritual growth, and social harmony are all linked to mind and body very intimately; therefore, they can be influenced through one medicine, if its knowledge goes deep enough. That is the argument Ayurveda advances—I think it is both profound and persuasive.

Characteristics of Vata Type

- Light, thin build
- Performs activity quickly
- Irregular hunger and digestion
- Light, interrupted sleep, insomnia
- Enthusiasm, vivaciousness, imagination
- Excitability, changing moods
- Quick to grasp new information, also quick to forget
- Tendency to worry
- Tendency toward constipation
- Tires easily, tendency to overexert
- Mental and physical energy comes in bursts

The basic theme of the Vata type is "changeable." Vata people are unpredictable and much less stereotyped than either Pittas or Kaphas, but their variability—in size, shape, mood, and action—is also their trademark. For a Vata person, mental and physical energy come in bursts, without steadiness. It is very Vata to:

- Be hungry at any time of the day or night
- Love excitement and constant change
- Go to sleep at different times every night, skip meals, and keep irregular habits in general
- Digest food well one day and poorly the next
- Display bursts of emotion that are short-lived and quickly forgotten
- Walk quickly

Physically, Vatas are the thinnest of the three types, with characteristically narrow shoulders and/or hips. Some Vatas may find it difficult or impossible to gain weight and remain chronically underweight; others are pleasingly slender and supple. Though they have quite variable appetites, Vatas are the only type who can eat anything without gaining weight. (Some Vatas, however, fluctuate widely in weight over their lifetimes; they may be rangy and weedy as adolescents but overweight in middle age.)

Physical irregularity comes from an excess of Vata—hands and feet may be too large for a given body, or too small; teeth may be very small or else large and protruding; having an overbite is a Vata characteristic. Although most Vata people are well shaped, bowlegs, pigeon-toes, spinal curvature (scoliosis), deviated septum, and eyes placed too close together or too far apart are also common. Bones may be either very light or very long and heavy. Joints, tendons, and veins stand out prominently on many Vata bodies because the layer of fat beneath the skin is thin. Cracking joints are considered highly typical.

Vata dosha is responsible for all movement in the body. Your muscles move because of Vata, which also controls breathing, the movement of food through the digestive tract, and nerve impulses emanating from the brain. Vata's most important function is to control the central nervous system. Tremors, seizures, and spasms are examples of Vata becoming disturbed. When this dosha is out of balance, nervous disorders appear, ranging from anxiety and depression (a hollow kind of depression, with feelings of being depleted, not the heavy depression of Kapha) to clinical mental disorders. Psychosomatic symptoms of all kinds are traceable to Vata aggravation. Therefore, bringing Vata back into balance often cures symptoms that defy any other treatment.

Vata is responsible for starting things, not finishing them, a characteristic that shows up strongly when a Vata type is out of balance—such people shop compulsively without buying anything, talk without coming to a conclusion, and become chronically unsatisfied. Vata types are sometimes said to spend themselves too freely, wasting money, energy, and words, but this is not true if they are in balance, since Vata dosha is responsible for balance throughout the body.

Most Vata people are prone to worry and at times suffer from insomnia, the result of restless thinking. Normal Vata sleep is the shortest of any type—six hours or less is characteristic, growing shorter as one ages. The typical negative emotion brought out by stress is anxiety (fear). The typical digestive complaint is chronic constipation and/or gas, although Vata people can also have nervous stomachs and unreliable digestion in general. Digestive cramps, as well as premenstrual pain, are generally attributed to this dosha.

A balanced Vata person is infectiously happy, enthusiastic, and energetic. The mind is clear and alert; the inner tone is exhilarated. Vatas are extremely sensitive to change in their environment. They have quick, acute responses to sound and touch and dislike loud noise. Personalities that are vivacious, vibrant, excitable, unpredictable, imaginative, and talkative all express Vata.

When out of balance, the Vata tendency to impulsiveness causes such people to overexert themselves—their excitement turns to exhaustion, then to chronic fatigue or depression.

Of all its qualities, perhaps the most important is that Vata leads the other doshas. This means several things: Vata goes out of balance first, causing the early stages of disease; it can mimic the other doshas, making you think that Pitta or Kapha is causing a problem (in fact, more than half of all disorders are Vata in origin); and it is "king" among the doshas, because when it is in balance, Pitta and Kapha generally are, too. Balancing Vata dosha, therefore, is vitally important for everyone.

The basic caution for Vata types is to get sufficient rest, not to overdo, and to pay close attention to regular lifestyle habits. These measures may not seem natural to many Vatas, but they often lead to quick improvements in physical or mental problems. We get our basic instinct for balance from Vata, which is absolutely vital to preserve.

Characteristics of Pitta Type

- Medium build
- Medium strength and endurance
- Enterprising character, likes challenges
- Sharp intellect
- Sharp hunger and thirst, strong digestion
- Tendency toward anger, irritability under stress
- Fair or ruddy skin, often freckled
- Aversion to sun, hot weather
- Precise, articulate speech
- Cannot skip meals
- Blond, light brown, or red hair (or reddish undertones)

The theme of the Pitta type is "intense." Anyone with bright red hair and a florid face contains a good deal of Pitta, as does anyone who is ambitious, sharp-witted, outspoken, bold, argumentative, or jealous. The combative side of Pitta is a natural tendency, but it does not have to be expressed. When in balance, Pittas are warm and ardent in their emotions, loving, and content. A face glowing with happiness is very Pitta. It is also very Pitta to:

- Feel ravenously hungry if dinner is half an hour late
- Live by your watch (generally an expensive one) and resent having your time wasted
- Wake up at night feeling hot and thirsty
- Take command of a situation or feel that you should
- Learn from experience that others find you too demanding, sarcastic, or critical at times
- Have a determined stride when you walk

Physically, Pittas are medium in size and well proportioned. They maintain their weight without drastic fluctuations; it is not difficult for them to gain or lose a few pounds at will. Facial features are well proportioned; eyes are medium in size, often with a penetrating glance. Hands and feet are medium, too; joints are normal.

Pitta hair and skin are easily recognizable. The hair is usually straight and fine, red, blond, or sandy in color, and tends to gray prematurely. Baldness, thinning hair, or a receding hairline is also a sign of strong or excess Pitta. The skin is warm, soft, and fair; it does not tan easily and often burns without tanning at all (particularly if the hair is fair and fine)—this gives Pittas another reason to stay out of the sun, which is their natural bent. It is also highly typical for Pitta skin to be marked with many freckles and moles. (In racial groups where dark hair and skin are the norm, other Pitta characteristics should be relied upon.)

Pittas generally have sharp, penetrating intellects and good powers of concentration. Their innate tendency is to be orderly and to manage their energies, money, and actions efficiently. Spending money on luxuries is one prominent exception to this—Pittas love to have fine things around them. They tend to respond to the world visually.

Heat is expressed everywhere in Pittas: by their typically short temper (hot-headedness), warm hands and feet, and burning sensations in the eyes, skin, stomach, or intestines— these are likely to appear if Pitta goes out of balance. Because they are hot themselves, Pittas are averse to long exposure to the sun. They develop heat fatigue very readily and do not take to hard physical labor. Their eyes dislike bright light.

Pittas incline toward anger as their characteristic negative emotion, and stress easily brings this out. They can be irritable and impatient, demanding and perfectionistic, particularly if out of balance. Although they are ambitious and show good leadership qualities, Pittas can be cutting and abrasive in manner, which alienates others.

Pittas speak precisely and articulately; they often make good public speakers. They hold strong opinions and like to argue. Sarcastic, critical speech identifies a Pitta imbalance, but, like people of the other doshas, Pitta types have two sides: in balance, they are sweet, joyous, confident, and brave. They like challenges and meet them vigorously, but with only medium physical energy. Pittas' stamina is moderate, and even their extremely strong digestion, the basis of their energy, can be abused. They are the kind of people who in middle age tend to say, "I used to be able to eat anything, but not anymore."

Pitta dosha controls metabolism in all body types. In Pitta people, the "digestive fire," as Ayurveda calls it, is particularly strong. This gives Pittas a large appetite for food and often excessive thirst. Of all the body types, Pittas are least able to skip a meal or even to eat late—it makes them feel ravenous and/or irritable. Excess Pitta is associated with heartburn, a tendency toward stomach ulcers, burning sensations in the intestine, and hemorrhoids. If not attended to, aggravated Pitta will seriously weaken the digestion.

Pitta skin tissue is easily irritated, causing rashes, inflammation, and acne. The whites of Pitta eyes are sensitive and turn red easily (poor eyesight also tends to be associated with Pitta imbalance). Pittas sleep soundly but may wake up during the night feeling overheated. They sleep a moderate length of time and come closest to the "normal" eight hours a night. If out of balance, Pittas suffer from insomnia, particularly if they are wrapped up in their work, which tends to be all-consuming for them.

The basic caution for a Pitta type is to lead a moderate, pure lifestyle. Every cell in the body relies on Pitta dosha to regulate its intake of pure food, water, and air. Toxins of all types show up quickly as Pitta imbalance. Being especially sensitive to this, Pitta types respond badly to impure food, polluted air and water, alcohol and cigarettes, and especially to toxic emotions—hostility, hatred, intolerance, jealousy. Pitta dosha gives us our instinct for moderation and purity, qualities that are vital to health.

Characteristics of Kapha Type

- Solid, powerful build; great physical strength and endurance

- Steady energy; slow and graceful in action
- Tranquil, relaxed personality; slow to anger
- Cool, smooth, thick, pale, often oily skin
- Slow to grasp new information, but good retentive memory
- Heavy, prolonged sleep
- Tendency to obesity
- Slow digestion, mild hunger
- Affectionate, tolerant, forgiving
- Tendency to be possessive, complacent

The basic theme of the Kapha type is "relaxed." Kapha dosha, the structural principle in the body, brings stability and steadiness; it provides reserves of physical strength and stamina that have been built into the sturdy, heavy frames of typical Kapha people. Kaphas are considered fortunate in Ayurveda because as a rule they enjoy sound health; moreover, their personalities express a serene, happy, tranquil view of the world. It is very Kapha to:

- Mull things over for a long time before making a decision
- Wake up slowly, lie in bed a long time, and need coffee once you are up
- Be happy with the status quo and preserve it by conciliating others
- Respect other people's feelings, with which you feel genuine empathy
- Seek emotional comfort from eating
- Have graceful movements, liquid eyes, and a gliding walk, even if overweight

Physically, Kapha dosha gives strength and natural resistance to disease. Besides being well built, Kapha types tend to be thickset, with wide hips and/or shoulders. There is a strong tendency to gain weight easily—Kaphas have only to look at food to put on a few pounds. Since extra weight is not easily lost, Kaphas often become obese when they are out of balance. However, people with moderate builds can still be Kapha, and in two-dosha types, such as Vata-Kapha, the body can even be thin. A telltale Kapha trait is cool, smooth, thick, pale skin that is often oily. Large, soft, doelike eyes ("as if filled with milk," the ancient texts say) are also highly typical. Anything about the face or the body shape that suggests repose and stability points to an underlying dominance of Kapha. In women, to have a full, curvaceous shape or statuesque Renaissance beauty is very Kapha.

Kapha dosha is slow. Slow eaters, who usually have slow digestion, are generally Kapha types, as are slow speakers, particularly if their speaking manner is deliberate. Being calm and self-contained, Kapha types are slow to anger and want to maintain peace around themselves. Their natural response to the world is through taste and smell—Kaphas tend to place a great deal of importance on food; in a more general way, they rely on bodily feelings, being essentially earthy people.

Kaphas have steady energy. Their stamina exceeds that of other types, as does their willingness to perform physical labor. They are rarely drained by physical fatigue. It is very Kapha to store and save almost everything—money, possessions, energy, words, food, and fat. The fat is usually stored lower down, in the thighs and buttocks.

Because this dosha controls the moist tissues of the body, a Kapha imbalance will tend to show up in the mucous membranes. Kaphas complain of sinus congestion, chest colds, allergies, asthma, and painful joints (although arthritis is typically Vata-related). These symptoms are worst in late winter and spring.

By nature Kaphas are affectionate, tolerant, and forgiving; to be motherly is to express Kapha. Kaphas are not easily shaken in a crisis, and they anchor others around them. There is a tendency to be complacent, however, and even the most balanced Kapha will procrastinate if he feels stressed. The typical Kapha negative emotion is greed or overattachment. Anyone who cannot bear to throw out old things is expressing an excess of Kapha. When out of balance, Kapha types become stubborn, dull, lethargic, and lazy.

Along with Vata, Kapha is a cold dosha, but it differs from Vata in not being dry. Since their circulation is generally good, Kapha types do not complain of cold hands and feet. They dislike cold, damp weather and respond to it mentally by becoming slower or outright depressed. Kapha sleep is long and heavy. Typical Kaphas often sleep more than eight hours a night; their common sleep disorder is not insomnia but oversleep. After taking a long time to get started in the morning, they feel energetic until late at night.

Of the three doshas, Kaphas are the slowest learners, but, in compensation, they have good retention and in time acquire a solid command of their subject. They absorb new information slowly and take a methodical approach to it. Out of balance, they become dull and thickheaded.

The basic caution for Kapha types is to progress. Any stagnant situation turns Kapha stability into inertia—Kapha types need to make sure that they do not hold on to the past, cling to people and possessions, or balk at change. Making sure that they have a good deal of stimulation, though not natural to many Kaphas, brings out their vitality; heavy, cold food, lack of exercise, overeating, and repetitive work do not. Kapha dosha gives us a sense of inner security and steadiness, an essential aspect of a healthy person.

UNDERSTANDING A TWO-DOSHA TYPE

Everyone is endowed at birth with some of each dosha. What makes it possible to describe "pure" Vatas, Pittas, or Kaphas is that they have so much of one dosha—they are extremes. This is not true of most people, however. Most people are two-dosha types, with one dosha predominant but not extreme.

The minority who are single-dosha types are fortunate in a sense, because they have to pay attention to only one dominant factor in their lives. However, this advantage is minor. *Everyone needs to balance all three doshas.* Although you will naturally pay closest attention to your own body type, being familiar with all the doshas makes a lot of sense. The best way to think of any body type is that all three doshas are expressing themselves, but one or two get the lion's share of attention.

In brief, the telltale signs of the three pure body types are:

Vata: Thin body, quick, changeable mind, vivacious manner. These people strike others as unpredictable. Under pressure they grow excited and anxious.

Pitta: Medium body, orderly and decisive mind, forceful manner. These people strike others as intense. Under pressure they become angry and abrupt.

Kapha: Heavyset body, calm, steady mind, easygoing manner. These people strike others as relaxed. Under pressure they balk and grow silent.

You can couple these sets of characteristics and arrive at a good approximation of what a two-dosha person is like. A Vata-Kapha, for instance, can be both excitable and calm, a seemingly unlikely combination that is quite obvious in these people. The dominant dosha gives a person his primary

reactions to the world, both physical and mental. The second
dosha exerts its influence in various ways—but as a rule the
two do not blend like colors of paint. If you combine Vata,
which produces a thin build, with Kapha, which produces a
heavy build, you do not generally get a medium build (a
medium build is distinctly Pitta). What actually happens is
that a Vata-Kapha type shows one trait or the other. Even so,
there are times when a person is clearly alternating from one
dosha to the other (a Pitta-Vata may tend toward both fear
and anger under stress, either together or at different times).

In Ayurvedic practice, we have observed the following
things about two-dosha types, which may help you to gain a
better understanding of how the three doshas combine.

VATA-PITTA

Generally these people are thin in build like the pure Vata
type. Like their Vata counterparts, they are quick-moving,
friendly, and talkative, but they tend to be more enterprising
and sharper of intellect (both Pitta traits). They are less likely
to approach the extremes of Vatas—they are not as high-strung
or physically fragile and/or irregular. Their constitution gains
overall stability from the influence of Pitta. Generally they also
have stronger digestion than Vata types and greater tolerance
for cold, since Pitta improves the circulation. Pure Vata types,
who are extremely sensitive to their environment, often
become prey to their intolerance of noise, cold drafts, and
physical discomfort, but this is less true of Vata-Pittas.

PITTA-VATA

People with this body type tend to have a medium build;
they are stronger and more muscular than Vata-Pittas, who
come closer to the sinewy, bony physique of pure Vatas. Pitta-

Vatas are quick in their movements, have good stamina, and are often assertive. Pitta intensity is obvious in them. Vata's lightness is present, but less so. They have stronger digestion and more regular elimination than Vata-Pittas or Vatas. They welcome challenge and tackle problems enthusiastically and often aggressively.

Vata-Pitta and Pitta-Vata types may experience a tendency toward both fear and anger, the negative emotions of the two doshas. If they are out of balance and under stress, this combination makes them tense, hard-driven, and insecure. If there is an Ayurvedic type who exhibits the Type A behavior that cardiologists warn against, it would be the imbalanced Pitta-Vata, with Vata-Pitta a hair's-breadth behind.

PITTA-KAPHA

Kapha is such a strong structural element that it lends its thick, heavier physique to two-dosha types, even when it does not come first. Pitta-Kaphas are generally recognizable because they have Pitta intensity in their manner and a solid Kapha body. They are more muscular than Pitta-Vatas and may even be quite bulky. Their personalities may demonstrate Kapha stability but Pitta force, complete with a tendency toward anger and criticism, is usually far more evident than anything like Kapha serenity. This is a particularly good body type for athletes since it gives Pitta's energy and drive to Kapha's endurance. This type finds it hard to miss a meal. The combination of strong Pitta digestion and Kapha resistance generally gives excellent physical health.

KAPHA-PITTA

The structural solidity of Kapha will come out even more in this type. Kapha-Pittas tend to have good musculature but with a higher ratio of fat than Pitta-Kaphas or Pittas. They tend to look rounder in face and body as a result. They tend to move slower and be more relaxed than Pitta-Kaphas; their added Kapha gives even more stamina and steady energy. They feel good if they exercise regularly, offsetting Kapha's tendency toward inertia and dullness, but they are less motivated to be active than are Pitta-Kaphas.

VATA-KAPHA

This type often has quite a hard time identifying itself from a written test because Vata and Kapha tend to be opposites (not to mention the Vata tendency to be indecisive). Usually the giveaway is that a thin Vata frame is strikingly combined with Kapha's relaxed, easygoing manner, something no pure Vata ever displays. To view it another way, these are Kapha personalities who somehow did not acquire physical bulk. In fact, since Vata's irregularity dominates the physique, they can even be quite small.

Unlike Vatas, who are always in motion, Vata-Kaphas project a sense of inner stability; they tend to be even-tempered but can show Vata's alarmed reactions under stress. This type tends to be quick and efficient when action is called for, but they are aware of their Kapha tendency to procrastinate. The desire to store and save may also be present. Since both doshas are cold, they tend to strongly dislike cold weather. Their cold doshas can also give them irregular or slow digestion.

KAPHA-VATA

This type is close to Vata-Kapha but often more solidly built and slower moving. Kapha makes them even-tempered and probably more relaxed than Vata-Kaphas, without the strong Vata streak of enthusiasm. They also tend to be more athletic and to have greater stamina. As with Vata-Kaphas, they may complain of digestive irregularities and be intolerant of cold.

UNDERSTANDING A THREE-DOSHA TYPE

A three-dosha type is sometimes said to start off with the best chance for remaining in balance, because the ratio of Vata, Pitta, and Kapha is nearly even. There isn't one strong horse pulling the whole team. A true *Sama dosha prakruti* (balanced dosha body type) will tend to have lifelong good health, ideal immunity, and longevity. On the other hand, it is also held that once imbalances start to occur, three-dosha types have a disadvantage, because they have to pay attention to getting all three back into line (there is no lead horse to stop the team when it runs away).

The doshas like to shift, and there are so many thousands of ways for them to relate to one another that to be in equal ratio at birth is extremely improbable—it is like throwing three pennies on the ground and finding that they line up in a perfectly straight line. So you may be a two-dosha type after all. The important thing is not to fit a category but to learn about yourself, and this is possible even when your body type at first seems a little vague, as the three-dosha type tends to be.

CHAPTER 3

THE THREE DOSHAS— MAKERS OF REALITY

When an Ayurvedic doctor looks at you, he sees signs of the three doshas everywhere, but he cannot literally see the doshas themselves. Doshas are invisible. They govern the physical processes in your body without being quite physical themselves. We have called them "metabolic principles," a term that is quite abstract. Yet the doshas are concrete enough to be moved around, increased, and decreased; they can get "stuck" in tissues and displaced to parts of the body where they don't belong—so they are on the borderline of being physical. Lying as they do in the gap between mind and body, they resemble nothing that exists in our Western scientific framework. Vata, Pitta, and Kapha only come into clear focus once you begin to view yourself from an Ayurvedic perspective.

LEARNING TO "SEE" THE DOSHAS

Imagine that you are watching a color television picture. The screen appears to be filled with people, trees, animals, sky, and clouds, but on closer examination one is actually seeing just three kinds of dots, or phosphors—red, green, and blue—constantly shifting to form new images. Depending on how closely you look, you can see either the images or the dots. Both perspectives are valid, but the three dots are more fundamental. When the picture goes bad, they are what you need to adjust. Vata, Pitta, and Kapha are the three kinds of "dots" an Ayurvedic doctor sees in you. Your liver, kidneys, heartbeat, insulin level, and so on are patterns formed by the shifting interplay of the three doshas. And adjusting the body, like adjusting the TV picture, comes down to realigning the doshas in their ever-changing relationship to one another.

The way you approach any problem depends a lot on how you see it in the first place. Right now, you may not see your compulsive worrying in terms of unbalanced Vata or your uncontrollable temper in terms of excess Pitta. But given a slight shift of emphasis, you could, and then by adjusting Vata or Pitta, these problems could be more easily handled. Even as physical a thing as gaining weight depends on the invisible, all-pervasive influence of the doshas.

When you eat a large bowl of chocolate ice cream, you may think that the fat in it is what causes you to gain weight. In a strictly literal sense this is true, but the deeper cause lies within your doshas. To begin with, they determine whether you are hungry. They determine whether ice cream appeals to you rather than carrots or celery. And to a great extent they even determine whether the calories put on fat. Vata-type people convert more calories into energy and will therefore gain less weight from ice cream than Kapha types, who convert a higher percentage of their calories into body fat.

Without the doshas' input, the ice cream would not even get to your lips, much less to your cells. So the calories in chocolate ice cream play only a partial role in what happens to that food. The real director of your diet is your own inner intelligence, operating out of sight at a deeper level than calories.

The same holds for every other part of your life. It isn't cigarettes that cause lung cancer but the people who smoke them,
motivated by habits (or addictions) that have been trained into
their doshas over time. In a very real sense it is not you that
craves nicotine but your Vata, in its role as supervisor of the
nervous system. When the decision is made to stop smoking,
however, it *is* you that makes it, using the freedom of choice
that goes beyond your doshas.

Ayurvedic physicians are trained to hone in on the doshas
in order to "see" imbalances at the earliest possible stage. One
of the classical ways to assess the state of someone's doshas is
through pulse diagnosis. Doctors who have studied and practiced this technique for many years are often able to perceive
imbalances that are not obvious to the more casual observer.

Recently, a *vaidya* (Ayurvedic doctor) on our Chopra Center
faculty was evaluating a man who had come for a wellness
evaluation. During the interview, the man denied problems in
any aspect of his health. His sleep was sound, his digestion
was strong, and his elimination was regular. Other than the
usual stresses of a busy life, he considered himself completely
healthy.

As part of a complete physical examination, the Ayurvedic
doctor took the man's pulse. Within seconds of palpating his
wrist, the doctor asked, "How long have you been having
canker sores?" The man almost fainted with surprise, exclaim-
ing, "I forgot to mention that I had problems with canker
sores. It's the one health concern that I haven't been able to
eliminate."

The vaidya then went on to describe the state of the man's
doshas, explaining that the Pitta imbalances he was perceiving
in the pulse made it very likely his canker sores would be a
recurrent problem if he did not change his diet. He encouraged the man to reduce his intake of sour and fermented

foods, including yogurt and alcohol. Yogurt is not a good food for Pitta types, because it aggravates that dosha, as do all sour or fermented foods. Such dietary mistakes, combined with alcohol consumption and other Pitta-provoking influences, had led to this man's intermittent imbalance. By Western standards he had been healthy except for the occasional annoying mouth sores. By Ayurvedic standards, he had been courting imbalances that sooner or later had to be expressed.

Advising the man to reduce his intake of sour foods such as yogurt, aged cheese, vinegar, and tomatoes could help to reduce the imbalances that gave rise to his canker sores. Seeing yourself in terms of your doshas can provide a quick, accurate assessment of your health.

Besides being located in every cell, the three doshas are situated at major sites around the body. Each dosha has a primary location, known as its seat, which serves as a focal point for treatment.

If a dosha is starting to go out of balance, the first symptom will often occur at its seat. Intestinal gas, pain, or constipation is a typical symptom of aggravated Vata; an uncomfortably hot or painful sensation in the upper abdomen often indicates aggravated Pitta; chest congestion, cough, or a cold points to aggravated Kapha.

This does not mean that the first symptoms of imbalance always show up in these sites. An imbalance of Vata may disclose itself as lower-back pain or menstrual cramps (you will note, though, that these symptoms still focus attention on the lower torso, in the region of the colon). Since every dosha is present in all parts of the body, Vata imbalance can also migrate and show up as a headache, muscle cramp, asthma, or any of dozens of other symptoms.

Viewing illness as a problem of dosha imbalance makes prevention much more specific, since you know your body type's

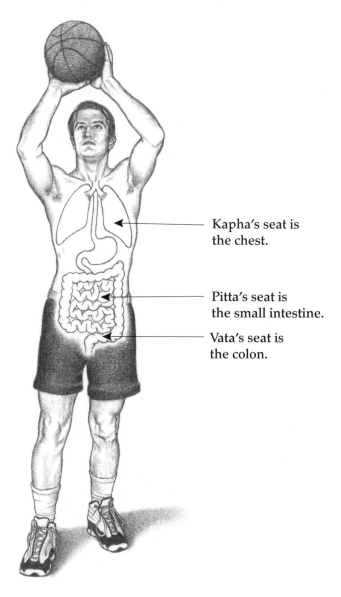

Kapha's seat is
the chest.

Pitta's seat is
the small intestine.

Vata's seat is
the colon.

Each dosha has a principal location or seat.

particular strengths and weaknesses. These tend to be permanent, or at least long-lasting. It is a rare Vata person who has
escaped insomnia his entire life, and Kapha types learn early

that they convert calories into body fat extremely easily. But what is really important is the knowledge that all sickness can be prevented, not by meticulously adjusting Vata, Pitta, and Kapha one at a time, but by balancing the whole system using the doshas as your guide.

BALANCE IS DYNAMIC—THE 25 GUNAS

Because they are intimately connected, the three doshas move together; even when you think you are working on just one, the others will respond, too. If you eat a bowl of hot chili, Pitta, the hot dosha, goes up, while the cold doshas, Vata and Kapha, go down. A drink of cold water brings Pitta down again, but it raises Vata and Kapha. They can be brought down by eating a little fennel seed, but that raises Pitta once more, and so on. The doshas are connected endlessly, in the ebb and flow typical of living things.

Vata stands out in capital letters (see below) because it changes first and drags the other two with it. This means that balancing the doshas is not like balancing the scales of justice

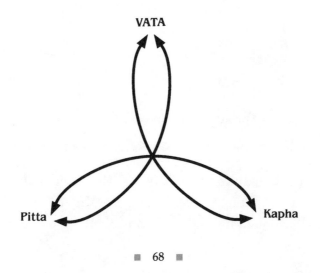

until things are equal. It is more like adjusting the flow of images on a TV set, as we mentioned. In other words, the doshas are balanced when they are in dynamic equilibrium. Change and permanence must be allowed interplay. To help achieve this state, Ayurveda describes certain enduring qualities evident throughout nature. There are twenty-five of these *gunas,* or fundamental qualities:

VATA	PITTA	KAPHA
Dry	Hot	Heavy
Moving	Sharp	Cold
Cold	Light	Oily
Light	Moist	Sweet
Changeable	Slightly Oily	Steady
Subtle	Fluid	Slow
Rough	Sour-smelling	Soft
Quick		Sticky
(Leads other doshas)		Dull
		Smooth

These gunas are consistent in nature, whether you are speaking of the world at large or the human body in particular. The heart is quick and moving—it contains Vata. Digestion and metabolism generate heat—they express Pitta. The mucous membranes are sticky and soft—they express Kapha.

THE DOSHAS AND THEIR QUALITIES

The twenty-five qualities, or gunas, are the source of all the characteristics we associate with each body type. Below are some of the leading qualities of Vata, Pitta, and Kapha, along with a few of the typical characteristics they produce.

VATA
Vata dosha is notably:

Cold, leading to cold hands and feet, dislike of cold climates.

Moving, giving good or bad circulation, depending on how well balanced this dosha is—hypertension is related to excess Vata, as are irregular heart rhythms, muscle spasms, and backaches. A nervous, darting glance is a sign of imbalanced Vata.

Quick, leading to many related characteristics: ability to pick up new information quickly, which is also quickly forgotten; poor long-term memory; good imagination but frightening dreams; restless activity; acting on impulse; mood swings; racing, scattered thoughts; and fast speech.

Dry, leading to dry skin, dry or dull hair, dull eyes, and scant or moderate sweat. Skin may chap and crack easily and be subject to psoriasis or eczema.

Rough, leading to rough skin and coarse-textured hair.

PITTA
Pitta dosha is notably:

Hot, leading to warm, flushed skin, any kind of inflammation or overactive metabolism, hot sensations in stomach, liver, intestines, and so on. Pittas are usually fond of cold food and drinks, which offset their own heat.

Sharp, leading to a sharp mind but also sharp speech; the same quality can turn into excess acidity in the body and oversecretion of stomach acids.

Moist, which may show up as profuse perspiration—hot, sweaty palms are typically Pitta. Being hot and moist gives Pittas an aversion to humid summer weather.

Sour-smelling, giving rise to bad breath, sour body odor, or bad-smelling urine and feces if excess Pitta is present.

KAPHA
Kapha dosha is notably:

Heavy. Any heavy disorder suggests Kapha imbalance, whether it is obesity, heavy digestion, or a heavy, oppressive kind of depression.

Sweet, leading to weight gain or diabetes if too much sweetness is added to the body.

Steady, which makes Kapha types self-contained. Bodily processes do not swing to extremes; Kapha's steady nature also has to do with not needing outside stimulation as much as Pitta or Vata. Their bodies remain unaffected by changes that would throw other body types out of balance.

Soft, leading to a wide variety of characteristics, such as soft skin and hair, soft manners, a soft look in the eyes, and an undemanding approach to situations.

Slow, as expressed in the typically slow, fluid movements of Kapha people, along with slow speech and deliberate thinking.

Dry, hot, and heavy are three good markers for the doshas. When anything becomes dry, Vata increases, whether it is a dry climate, the dry wind of autumn, or dry food (popcorn, crackers, dried prunes). If your skin or sinuses get too dry, then Vata is on the rise and probably going out of balance.

Anything hot increases Pitta. A hot day in July, a hot bath, and "hot" emotions like anger or sexual passion share this quality. If you feel burning sensations anywhere in your body (stomach, intestines, rectum) or your skin becomes inflamed, Pitta is rising. Pitta is not as subtle or penetrating as Vata; it is aggressive and sharp.

Anything that becomes heavy increases Kapha. Gaining weight, feeling heavy inside, or a heavy, overcast day will all cause more Kapha dosha to come out. If your sleep becomes much heavier than usual or makes you feel groggy instead of refreshed, then likely too much Kapha is to blame. Of all the doshas, Kapha is the steadiest, the closest to material form.

From the Ayurvedic standpoint, the body's systems exist to balance these twenty-five gunas. All of us have to make our way through a world that balances hot and cold, heavy and light, rough and smooth conditions. Warm air masses pursue cold arctic fronts, droughts succeed floods, high tides replace low. The play of nature is the play of these things. Ayurveda says that we ourselves are a balanced ecology, perfectly matched to the one outside us—we too move through contrasts that make us feel light or heavy, hot or cold, steady or unsteady, smooth or rough.

As you begin to consider the gunas associated with a particular dosha, their dynamic balance becomes more complex. Life grows more interesting, but at the same time, remaining in balance is more of a challenge. This is how nature sharpens our individuality and fine-tunes our senses. For example, Pitta is moist as well as hot, so muggy summer conditions are more challenging to Pitta people than is dry heat. Typically, a Pitta type can stand the desert better than the tropics. But there is a deeper significance than that.

More than twenty thousand years ago, prehistoric men crossed the land bridge that then connected Alaska and northern Asia, migrating through every region from the Arctic north to Tierra del Fuego, almost touching the Antarctic. The same gene pool produced Eskimos (who live almost solely on whale blubber, seals, and fish), Mexican Indians (who live on corn and beans), and Amazonian Indians (who live on the animals and plants of the tropical rain forest). The DNA in all these people is nearly identical; the same cells, organs, enzymes, and hormones are at work. But each people has attuned itself to a different environment—their inner ecology has learned to adapt to the outer one. One fascinating fact about Eskimos, the Indians of northern Mexico, and the Indians of the Amazon basin is that none of these groups has any heart disease to speak of.

This represents almost a miracle of natural adaptation, for none of these people achieved their diet by thinking about it— they ate what was available to them and relied on their bodies to strike the proper balance. Until very recently, thinking about a diet of whale blubber would give a nutritionist shudders, because of the extraordinarily high amounts of cholesterol. Now we point to the fact that blubber contains newly discovered omega-3 fatty acids, which are said to thin the blood and prevent dangerous clots from forming in the coronary arteries.

This ostensibly explains why Eskimos manage to enjoy a heart-attack rate that is 3 percent of that in the continental United States. But does it really? Other indigenous people related to the Eskimos are not eating omega-3 fats, yet they are just as protected. Although they live in different worlds, each people has found a healthy balance with nature, both inner and outer.

Can we say the same for ourselves? There is nothing intrinsic to modern life that means we must succumb to the epidemic of heart disease afflicting the United States and almost every other industrialized country. Ayurveda would say that we simply need to shape our inner world to match the outer one we have built for ourselves.

The ultimate significance of the twenty-five gunas is that they extend human nature beyond the confines of the body. As a collection of cells, a human being stops at the frontier of his skin; as a collection of gunas, he blends into nature as a whole. For example, Kapha dosha is cold and moist, so on a cold, damp, December day, Kapha imbalance becomes much more likely. People might become more depressed on such days, as in fact they do. There is even a specific syndrome, the much-publicized SAD (seasonal affective disorder), that affects certain people by making them extremely depressed in the winter.

The cause of SAD, from a Western perspective, is a deficiency of sunlight reaching the pineal gland, causing elevated levels of the hormone melatonin. How the pineal gland realizes that winter is here remains a mystery, however, since it is buried deep inside the skull and has no access to light. Ayurveda would use a simpler principle to explain SAD: When Kapha increases outside, it also increases inside. Certain people—those vulnerable to Kapha imbalance—will become sick from this added Kapha, leading to depression. All of us will be affected by the increase, though, because we all have Kapha within us.

In Ayurveda, there is no mystery: A sliding scale of effects takes in every person, healthy or ill. The challenge is not how to fight winter depression but how to flow with the change of seasons. Nature has given us this challenge, and it has given us the ability to meet it. Every day nature asks, "Is your ecology in balance?" and every day you have to come up with an answer. In the final analysis, whether you are healthy or sick is nature's verdict on your ability to remain in balance with the world, with the constant play of the gunas. Balance is flexibility in the face of change; perfect balance is perfect flexibility in the face of constant change.

THE FIVE ELEMENTS

How did Ayurveda figure out that Vata is dry, Pitta hot, Kapha heavy? The answer is fascinating, for it reveals a complete and profound view of nature. Vata, Pitta, and Kapha are the body's fundamental principles. As such, they are abstract, even though they take material form in blood, bones, stomach linings, heartbeats, and breathing.

The idea that everything we see in nature—stars, trees, lions, roses—is basically abstract at first seems foreign. Yet, since Einstein derived his famous theorem $E = mc^2$, establishing that matter can also take the form of energy, the abstractness of nature has gradually become accepted. Conversely, the most abstract concepts in physics are being discovered to have physical form. The force of gravity, which is the Western equivalent for the guna called "heavy," is currently discussed in terms of physical particles (gravitons) that can be moved and stored like bricks, at least in theory.

In the West we are comfortable saying that nature is founded on two levels of abstraction, matter and energy. Energy is more abstract than matter in our scheme, but it can still flow from place to place, increase or diminish, and be stored (as electricity is stored in batteries). In the Ayurvedic scheme, there are also two levels of abstraction, and they too agree with the senses, although in a slightly different way. One level contains the three doshas; the other contains a set of principles called the five elements.

The five elements have something of both matter and energy in them. In order from most subtle to most gross, they are:

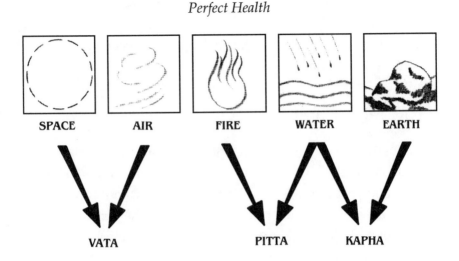

These elements correspond to "real" earth, air, fire, water, and space, but they are also abstract. Asked what the five elements represent, an Ayurvedic sage wouldn't point to the wind or a burning log or a brook. The five elements are a code for shapes of intelligence that make up man's mind and the world he perceives through that mind.

By mixing different pairs of the five elements, one arrives at the three doshas:

Vata is composed of air and space.
Pitta is composed of fire and water.
Kapha is composed of earth and water.

The connection between Vata imbalance and cold, windy weather is clearer now, because Vata is the "airy" dosha, and too much air, in the form of wind, creates too much Vata. A Vata person typically complains of gas in the intestines, showing that Vata and air are linked in another way. Air is subtle, penetrating, and light, as is Vata.

A Pitta person generally feels warm, showing his fire, and may be prone to sweating, showing the wateriness that is also in Pitta. Fire is aggressive, energetic, and mobile, as is Pitta.

A Kapha person is typically "down to earth" and prone to chest congestion, blocked sinuses, and other mucus problems, which are directly related to too much water. Together, water and earth are sluggish, viscous, and half-solid, half-liquid, as is the Kapha dosha.

The element of space, which seems odd in the company of the four elements you can see and feel, plays a unique role in the Ayurvedic system, because it allows the existence of sound, which needs space in order to travel. Sound is the basis of all existing things, according to Ayurveda, not audible sound like thunder but subtler vibrations that resonate in our silent awareness. Ayurveda uses such sounds to heal the body by moving its "vibrations" in various ways, which will be discussed more fully later.

After you spend a while using this new code, you will find that it is completely natural. All twenty-five gunas can be contacted by sight, touch, taste, and the other senses. The same cannot be said for enzymes, hormones, neurotransmitters, and the other building blocks of Western medicine. How many people do you know who can tell you the basic properties of insulin, for example? Yet in an hour you can easily learn the qualities of Kapha, the dosha which is most involved in balancing insulin.

GETTING DOWN TO DETAILS—THE SUBDOSHAS

For the sake of completion, I want to mention that each of the three doshas is broken down into five subdoshas, which make diagnosis and treatment more precise. All the subdoshas have their own locations in the body, giving rise to specific disorders when imbalances occur there. The most important subdosha of Vata, called Prana Vata, is situated in the upper chest and head, for example. It regulates the movement of breath and nerve impulses and therefore has a profound influence on every function in the body.

All three doshas have a subdosha sitting in the heart, which is an important crossroads for all physical and emotional activity in the body. Such detailed knowledge is essential for an Ayurvedic physician to know; it is optional for the patient. (For a complete description of the fifteen subdoshas, see the reference pages at the end of this chapter.) To show you how all this information about the doshas adds up, let's look at a case history.

Ann Holmes began to experience menstrual pain in her early teens; it became increasingly severe in adulthood. For nearly a week every month she was incapacitated by cramps, vomiting, and diarrhea. For a few days prior to her period she was nervous and upset in anticipation of what was coming; the week following left her feeling exhausted. Altogether, she was unable to work for as much as two weeks every month.

Her attempts to solve this problem ranged far and wide. One doctor recommended megadoses of vitamins. "My periods simply stopped coming," she recalls. "I was relieved to be free of pain, but I didn't feel that this was a cure. When I went back and told my doctor, he reduced the vitamins, but then the problem returned almost as bad as before."

Over a two-year period Ann saw several more specialists. A gynecologist put her on heavy doses of Motrin, a non-narcotic pain reliever that alleviated her symptoms somewhat. Other doctors agreed that she should stay on medication or turn to surgery.

"The pain had spread throughout my lower abdomen and back. I couldn't lift heavy objects or walk a long distance anymore, but at the same time, I knew that I didn't want any solution that involved a hysterectomy." Since past episodes had required hospitalization, Ann decided that she should adjust to her condition and be thankful that it was not totally debilitating. After several years without relief, however, she was discouraged enough to think that surgery was inevitable. At this point she consulted a physician trained in Ayurveda. His outlook was startling.

"He did not seem at all perplexed when I gave him my medical history. He described my pain in terms of what he called my doshas. I learned that Vata dosha was dominant in my body type, and when severely out of balance, Vata commonly causes menstrual difficulties. Pain in general is associated with imbalance of Vata. There is also a specific subdosha of Vata in the lower back and abdomen called Apana Vata that leads to muscle weakness and pain there. All in all, my symptoms presented a clear picture to him."

Ann was relieved to hear that her disease made sense. The absence of this reassurance had added considerably to her feelings of confusion and guilt. The Ayurvedic doctor proposed to wean her off medication by bringing Vata back into balance. This involved a change of diet, daily oil massage that put special emphasis on the abdomen, warm baths, hot milk in the evening, and careful attention to maintaining a regular routine. (Vata dosha responds quickly to all of these measures, as explained in detail in later chapters.)

Ann was also given an herb that helps to calm Vata and asked to return to the center for periodic physical purification, a routine called *panchakarma*. The purpose of panchakarma is to flush the toxic residues of past imbalances out of the body, an essential step for anyone who has reached the stage of overt illness. Except for this last therapy, everything Ann was asked to do could be done at home at nominal cost.

The results of treatment were excellent and improved over time. "The day I started Ayurveda, I was taking twenty 400-mg capsules of Motrin a day. Within a few months I was down to five capsules. I kept on my prescribed program and returned for panchakarma twice a year. Now, three years later, my periods last four days instead of a week. The pain and discomfort have decreased to the extent that I have taken no medication for the last ten months.

"It's absolutely a transformation to have my confidence return. I feel like a normal, happy person again, not like a martyr who has to view each month as a matter of survival."

THE SUBDOSHAS—A MORE PRECISE GUIDE

To locate the origin of disease as precisely as possible, an Ayurvedic doctor looks beyond the three doshas to their subdoshas. There are fifteen of these, covering every part of the body. The following reference information is provided to give you a more exact idea of how the doshas actually operate in daily life.

Vata

Vata is connected with the nervous system and therefore reaches every part of the body, but each of the five Vata subdoshas has an assigned location and function. Traditionally, Ayurveda also calls these the "winds" of the body, or as we would put it, the impulses traveling along nerves, muscles, blood vessels, anywhere there is bodily motion.

Prana Vata: located in brain, head, chest
Prana Vata is responsible for perception and movement of all kinds. Like the brain, where it is located, Prana Vata enables you to see, hear, touch, smell, and taste (but primarily to hear and touch); it enlivens the ability to think, reason, and feel and

gives tone to all emotions, positive and negative. In balance, it makes you alert, clearheaded, exhilarated, and lively. It also governs the rhythm of respiration and swallowing, and is considered upward-moving, hence its connection to higher functions.

Prana Vata is the "leader" of the other four subdoshas and the most important aspect of Vata dosha. Since Vata leads the body as a whole, Prana Vata is also considered the most important of all the subdoshas. Keeping it healthy is vital for every bodily function.

Imbalance of Prana Vata is linked to worry, anxiety, overactive mind, insomnia, neurological disorders, hiccups, asthma and other respiratory complaints, and tension headaches.

Udana Vata: located in throat and lungs

Physically, this subdosha controls the process of speech. Through the speech center in the brain, it is also responsible for memory and the movement of thought.

Imbalance of Udana Vata is linked to speech defects, dry coughs, sore throats, tonsilitis, earaches, and generalized fatigue.

Samana Vata: located in stomach and intestines

This subdosha controls the movement of food throughout the digestive tract; it is responsible for the rhythm of peristalsis.

Imbalance of Samana Vata is linked to too slow or too rapid digestion, gas, diarrhea, nervous stomach, inadequate assimilation of nutrients, and emaciated tissue formation.

Apana Vata: located in the colon and lower abdomen

This downward-moving subdosha is responsible for elimination of wastes and, outside the digestive tract, for sexual function and menstruation. One of its locations, the colon, is considered the principal seat of Vata and is the site where early signs of Vata imbalance are likely to originate.

Imbalance of Apana Vata is linked to constipation, diarrhea, gas, intestinal cramps, colitis, genito-urinary disorders, menstrual disorders, swollen prostate, various sexual dysfunctions, and lower back pain, including muscle spasm.

Vyana Vata: located throughout the body via the nervous system, skin, and circulatory system

This subdosha governs circulation in its diverse aspects, but particularly heart rhythm, dilation and constriction of the blood vessels, and peripheral circulation. Blood pressure is regulated by Vyana Vata; it is also responsible for sweating, yawning, and the sensation of touch.

Imbalance of Vyana Vata is linked to high blood pressure, poor circulation, irregular heart rhythm, and stress-related nervous disorders.

Pitta

Pitta is responsible for metabolism and is equated with the body's heat, as well as with digestion in general. Acuteness of sight and sharp thinking are also Pitta functions. There are five Pitta subdoshas, situated at various locations in the body.

Pachaka Pitta: located in stomach and small intestine

Pitta's seat is in the small intestine, making this an important subdosha. Pachaka Pitta is vital in its function of digesting food and separating nutrients from waste products. It also regulates the "heat" of digestion, making it fast or slow, efficient or weak. The appearance of foul smells during elimination or an inability properly to extract nourishment from your diet may be due to imbalance here.

Imbalance of Pachaka Pitta is linked to heartburn, aciu stomach, ulcers, and irregular digestion (either too weak or hyperactive).

Ranjaka Pitta: located in red blood cells, liver, spleen

The complex processes involved in producing healthy red blood cells, balancing blood chemistry, and distributing nutrients through the bloodstream are governed by this subdosha. The presence of toxicity in the body, from impure food, air, water, alcohol, or cigarettes, is considered a primary cause of Pitta imbalance, acting through Ranjaka Pitta.

Imbalance of Ranjaka Pitta is linked to jaundice, anemia, various blood disorders, skin inflammations, anger, and hostility.

Sadhaka Pitta: located in heart

Besides controlling the heart's physical function, Sadhaka Pitta creates contentment that comes from the heart, as we say; it is also associated with good memory. If you lack the heart to face challenges and make important decisions, this subdosha may be weak.

Imbalance of Sadhaka Pitta is linked to heart disease, memory loss, emotional disturbance (sadness, anger, heartache), and indecisiveness.

Alochaka Pitta: located in eyes

Sight is the primary sense related to Pitta dosha. Alochaka Pitta is the subdosha associated with good or bad vision, depending on its state of balance. It also connects the eyes with emotions; when you "see red," go "blind" with rage, or have an angry look in your eyes, Alochaka Pitta has become aggravated. In balance, it creates bright, clear, healthy eyes. A warm, content gaze shows very healthy Pitta.

Imbalance of Alochaka Pitta is linked to bloodshot eyes, vision problems, and eye diseases of all kinds.

Bhrajaka Pitta: located in the skin

Along with Vata dosha, our sensitivity to the world through our skin depends on Pitta, acting through this subdosha. It is very Pitta to have irritable, red, or inflamed skin. Pitta types blush easily and show their emotions through the skin, developing rashes, boils, and acne under conditions of stress. In balance, Bhrajaka Pitta gives a glowing complexion that radiates happiness and vitality.

Imbalance of Bhrajaka Pitta is linked to rashes, acne, boils, skin cancers, and skin disorders of all types.

Kapha

Kapha's five subdoshas complete the fifteen subdoshas in the body. The themes of Kapha are structure and moistness. These subdoshas are responsible for keeping tissues and joints soundly knit and well lubricated; the moist senses, taste and smell, are also governed by Kapha.

Kledaka Kapha: located in the stomach

This subdosha keeps the stomach lining moist and is essential for digestion. The stomach is an extremely important site of Kapha as a whole, since excessive buildup of this dosha often appears here first. In traditional Ayurveda, excess Kapha is removed by vomiting; this is not practiced at the Chopra Center, since it places too great a strain on the body. In balance, Kledaka Kapha gives a strong, supple, well-lubricated stomach lining.

Imbalance of Kledaka Kapha is linked to impaired digestion (usually too slow and heavy).

Avalambaka Kapha: located in heart, chest, and lower back

Kapha's seat is in the chest, so this is an important subdosha. Avalambaka Kapha keeps the chest, lungs, and back strong. A typical Kapha's physical stamina comes from these areas, so the Kapha physique usually exhibits a powerful chest and shoulders. In balance, Avalambaka Kapha provides strong muscles and protects the heart. Troubles develop when it goes out of balance, leading to chest congestion, wheezing, asthma, and congestive heart failure, depending on the seriousness of the imbalance. Under these conditions, Kapha types lose their accustomed energy and freedom from disease. Smoking is one of the worst insults to this critical subdosha.

Imbalance of Avalambaka Kapha is linked to respiratory problems of all types, lethargy, and lower back pain.

Bhodaka Kapha: located in the tongue

This subdosha allows us to perceive taste. Unlike Western medicine, Ayurveda gives great importance to taste as the guide for nutrition and also for the effects of medicine. Kaphas respond to the world primarily through taste, along with its companion sense, smell. In Kapha types who have abused the sense of taste, compulsive eating becomes a problem. The taste buds lose their sensitivity if you eat too much or too often. They are also desensitized by concentrating on only a few taste sensations. When taste goes, the body becomes much more liable to other Kapha problems, such as obesity, food allergies, congestion of mucous membranes, and diabetes.

Imbalance of Bhodaka Kapha is linked to impairment of taste buds and salivary glands.

Tarpaka Kapha: located in the sinus cavities, head, and spinal fluid

Keeping the nose, mouth, and eyes moist protects these sense organs; maintenance of spinal fluid is essential for the central nervous system. All of this is controlled by Tarpaka Kapha, which should be fluid and movable. When it goes out of balance, this subdosha becomes clogged or excessively runny, the two sides of typical Kapha sinus problems.

Imbalance of Tarpaka Kapha is linked to sinus congestion, hay fever, sinus headache, impaired sense of smell, and general dullness of senses.

Shleshaka Kapha: located in the joints

Through this subdosha, the only one that is not localized, Kapha lubricates every joint in the body. Most Kapha imbalances appear in the chest, spreading up to the head. The main exception is aching joints, which can appear anywhere. Too much Vata in a joint dries it out, creating arthritic symptoms; too much Pitta heats and inflames a joint, causing rheumatoid symptoms; too much Kapha creates loose or watery joints.

Imbalance of Shleshaka Kapha is linked to loose, watery, or painful joints and various joint diseases.

CHAPTER 4

A BLUEPRINT FROM NATURE

If you are ever stranded at an airport, observe how the people around you are reacting. Some will fret and rush around trying to find another flight, expressing a Vata tendency toward anxiety and impatience. Others will fume, blame the airlines for incompetence, and angrily demand that their tickets be honored, expressing a Pitta tendency toward anger and criticism. Still others will sit tight and refuse to budge, expressing a Kapha tendency toward resignation and staying put.

Feeling anxious, angry, or resigned is more than a mood. Each body type thinks its response is natural; the doshas color the situation and turn it into a convincing version of reality. Try to get an anxious Vata type to act patient and you will quickly learn how convincing that Vata's view of the world really is.

Of course, these stereotypes have their limits. Everyone has some Pitta; under enough pressure, it will be aroused and turn to anger. Similarly, fear is not limited to imbalanced Vata types, nor is staying put an exclusive property of Kaphas. Nonetheless, your innate tendencies will surface time and again, because that is how nature shaped you. The doshas provide so much information that calling your Ayurvedic type a body type is really too limited: it is a mind body type. Being mentally restless is just as Vata as being physically restless; to suffer from skin rashes or rash behavior is just as Pitta; to rise slowly to a conclusion or to the morning sun is just as Kapha.

Taken together, your doshas express your nature as a whole. Therefore, Ayurveda uses the Sanskrit word for nature, *prakruti*, to describe how each person is constituted from birth. Instead of saying, "Vata is my body type," you can substitute, "I have Vata prakruti"—the two are interchangeable. Having introduced this term a few chapters back, I now want to show how respecting your prakruti is the best way to tailor your plan for complete balance.

RESPECT YOUR BODY TYPE

By the time we are adults, most of us know our basic tendencies, but that does not mean we can do anything about them. Far from it. The same complaints often bother people for life. Once the seeds of depression, obesity, insomnia, or other chronic problems are sown, they seem to grow regardless of our desire *not* to be depressed, overweight, or sleepless. These problems grow out of our prakruti, and unless they are uprooted at that fundamental level they will continue to expand their influence, like noxious weeds choking out flowers in a garden.

Let's not think in terms of symptoms, however. Everyone needs to respect his prakruti in order to make life better, to rise to a higher state of health. This is one of the first lessons in learning how to be a balanced person. If you never learn it, higher realities are attainable only in glimpses.

Bobby Thomas was diagnosed as a pure Vata type, which certainly matches his naturally thin frame and his bright, outgoing personality. Bobby is the kind of person who flashes a smile at everyone he meets. Being quick and responsive, he decided that it would be easy for him to work his way through college waiting on tables, but the incessant demands of working in a crowded restaurant threw his Vata badly out of balance, making him feel restless and unhappy.

Bobby looked around at the other waiters, who seemed to be thriving in the environment, or at least treating it as no more stressful than any other work situation. "What's wrong with me?" Bobby wondered. He decided to work even harder. But this tactic failed utterly. He began to sleep badly. He lost his appetite and started losing weight. Within a few months, he was complaining of various aches and pains that seemed to have no physical cause.

Bobby came to the Chopra Center thinking he needed tranquilizers, and no doubt he would have gotten them fairly easily from most doctors, since he certainly looked anxious and unable to settle down. However, after a close examination, his Ayurvedic doctor told him, "From everything you've told me, it doesn't seem that you are actually sick." Bobby looked surprised, even offended. Weren't his symptoms as real as anybody else's? It was explained that what he was experiencing was a classic case of aggravated Vata. In Western medicine, each of his complaints would be neatly classified under textbook headings of "insomnia," "anxiety," "lower back pain," and so on. But if you traced these signals of distress back to their origin, only one thing was at fault—fundamental imbalance that cried out in different ways.

Fortunately, treating Vata is a lot simpler than trying to treat five or six symptoms. In Bobby's case, we didn't need to resort to medicine, because the diagnosis itself was enough. Rather than prescribing medications, which tend to mask the underlying problem, we suggested that he simply listen to his body.

It was suggested that his body type wasn't suited for the work he was in. He was encouraged to find a job that would make his Vata happy instead of driving it crazy. Whatever he did, Bobby was not going to adapt well to noise, overcrowding, and constant activity because his Vata couldn't tolerate it.

What does Vata actually like? A little more peace and quiet, for one thing. Bobby might be happier as a prep chef working when the restaurant kitchen is relatively quiet. Creativity is another thing that imaginative Vata types thrive on. A job that satisfies this deeper part of their nature will be much more satisfying in the long run. Once again, cooking might be good for Bobby, but so might performing, designing, or other work where self-expression is valued. Bobby took our advice. As soon as he quit the restaurant and got a little rest, his major symptoms disappeared. Within a few months he moved on to a job in graphic design and has not returned with any problems.

Making your doshas happy will make you happy. That is *the* secret to balancing the whole mind body system. To respect your body type, you have to trust that its needs are good for you. Telling Bobby to look for a new job was in line with what his body was already saying. No one can be happy or healthy in an unbalanced state, because it is just not natural.

AS NATURE MADE YOU

Like the doshas, your prakruti is double-edged. You can see yourself as trapped by it, or you can learn from it and benefit from what your system is trying to tell you. A Pitta nature may predispose you to hostility and a Vata nature to irritable bowels, but nothing forces you to embrace the stressful lifestyle that fans Pitta to a flame or drives Vata to exhaustion, bringing out such problems. Living with your doshas is a perfect example of how to find freedom within your nature's limits.

Because you were born with it, your body type does not change. On the other hand, the doshas are constantly in flux. Every time you look at a mountain, eat a potato chip, listen to Mozart, or carry out any thought or action, your doshas shift. A person whose heart is pounding is having a strong Vata reaction, no matter what his basic nature is. *Whatever your prakruti happens to be, try to live all three doshas fully.* To be completely healthy, everyone needs to experience and express the best that can be derived from each of the doshas—that is what it means to become a complete person.

The positive psychological traits of each dosha include the following:

Vata—imaginative, sensitive, spontaneous, resilient, exhilarated

Pitta—intellectual, confident, enterprising, joyous

Kapha—calm, sympathetic, courageous, forgiving, loving

Whenever you meet someone who lives up to all of these qualities, naturally you are impressed. Such a person has accepted the greatest gift of nature—perfect balance. Rare as it is, perfect balance is not abnormal; it is possible for everyone to achieve.

Every body type contains a wide range of possibilities. Unfortunately, we all have a tendency to compare ourselves to a norm, which generates feelings of inadequacy when we cannot live up to the standards we feel everyone must meet. Such conformity is not in nature's plan. Take the following example:

Body weight is a sensitive subject. Everyone wants to maintain an ideal weight, but millions of people struggle in vain. Critics point out that our society is obsessed with thinness at any price; women in particular feel anxious and unworthy if they don't look as if they just stepped out of the pages of *Vogue*. (The current fad for weight training has added a little more muscle to the desirable female frame, but it has also stripped acceptable body fat down to near zero.)

Ayurveda would say that the trouble does not lie in our fixation on the perfect figure but in ignorance about nature's underlying design. By nature, a Vata woman will be thin and a Kapha solid, if not actually heavy. What gives both types their undeniable attractiveness lies deeper. Vatas are charming, vivacious, and vibrant—they communicate a natural sense of exhilaration. Kaphas may not be blessed with light, agile bodies, but they have their own beauty—they are serene, with large, soft eyes, a graceful manner, and a full, gently contoured figure. In the eyes of an Ayurvedic doctor, this is the ideal type, as healthy as it is beautiful. Pittas, who come closest to our current Western notions of the ideal type physically, being medium in build and well proportioned, also have a quality of self-control that makes them attractive to others. Each dosha, then, provides an ideal that is of equal worth in nature's eyes; it should be equal in our eyes, too.

People sometimes think that "balancing the doshas" means trying to get equal amounts of Vata, Pitta, and Kapha. That is mistaken; you cannot change the ratio of doshas you were born with. What you can do is find the balance that is right for each dosha in you. The doshas function on a sliding scale, with too much or too little at either end of the scale and a point of balance in the middle:

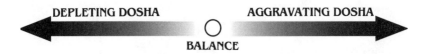

DEPLETING DOSHA   **AGGRAVATING DOSHA**

BALANCE

Ayurveda tells you to keep as close to the balance point as you can. This is not something you have to concentrate on. Your body keeps in balance by following its normal processes.

But since the doshas are so responsive to your habits, you do need to learn how to stop pulling them out of balance.

It is customary to think mainly in terms of aggravating a dosha rather than depleting it, because being a Vata, Pitta, or Kapha type indicates that you already have a good amount of that one dosha. Your aim is not to add more (aggravate the dosha), which would lead to imbalance. A Vata person who has developed weak digestion could be diagnosed as having depleted Pitta, but for all practical purposes he is treated as having aggravated Vata, the most likely cause of the problem.

If a dosha goes out of balance, you would typically notice the following physical symptoms:

Vata is unbalanced when there is pain, spasms, cramps, chills, or shakiness.

Pitta is unbalanced when there is inflammation, fever, excessive hunger and thirst, heartburn, or hot flashes.

Kapha is unbalanced when there is congestion, mucus discharge, heaviness, fluid retention, lethargy, or over-sleeping.

These simple guidelines can help you when you have unexplained symptoms of illness (a more detailed description of how to spot imbalances is given at the end of this chapter). We should emphasize that guidelines are not a substitute for medical school; an Ayurvedic physician, like his Western counterpart, spends a lifetime learning to diagnose disorders of all kinds. Any dosha can give rise to any symptom. Constipation, a textbook sign of Vata imbalance, can be due to Pitta or Kapha in some cases; this holds true for every other typical symptom. If you are seriously ill, you need a professional opinion about your condition.

When symptoms turn into chronic conditions, diagnoses based on body types continue to be useful. Vata, Pitta, and

Kapha people tend to be susceptible to different disorders, both physical and mental.

Vata types are prone to insomnia, chronic constipation, nervous stomach, anxiety and depression, muscle spasms or cramps, PMS (premenstrual syndrome), irritable bowel, chronic pain, high blood pressure, and arthritis.

Pitta types are prone to rashes, acne, heartburn, peptic ulcers, early balding and premature gray hair, poor eyesight, hostility, self-criticism, and heart attacks related to stress (Type A behavior).

Kapha types are prone to obesity, congested sinuses, chest colds, painful joints, asthma and/or allergies, depression, diabetes, high cholesterol, and chronic sluggishness in the morning.

This simply outlines the broad shape of things. There is no simple one-to-one relationship between a disease and a body type. Being a Vata does not mean that nature has doomed you to get arthritis, nor does being a Pitta or a Kapha automatically protect you from it. Illness is individual and depends on the overall pattern of your life, with body type serving as an important influence, not a cause.

Also, major disorders such as heart disease and cancer are the result of more than one dosha becoming unbalanced. Once one dosha is disturbed, the others will follow suit unless balance is restored. Although different in severity, colds and asthma are linked in Ayurveda, because they often involve Vata going out of balance first, followed by Kapha aggravation. Knowing the dosha that usually leads the pack (it is usually Vata) helps you to correct the imbalance as soon as possible. When you see someone who is angry and anxious at the same time, a typical combination in high-stress situations, you quickly recognize that Vata has gone out of balance and led Pitta after it.

You will notice that some of the symptoms of dosha imbalance are mental. This is an important fact. *Your mind first detects imbalances in the body.* Since a balanced body makes the mind alert, clear, sensitive, and happy, its absence causes these qualities to decline. When they do, something has gone wrong with a dosha. By standards accepted in our society, you can be normal without being happy. Ayurveda argues that this is not nature's standard of health, however; unhappiness indicates that action is needed now to avoid disease in the future.

THE SUBTLE SOURCE OF DISEASE

Recently we saw a woman who had undergone a mastectomy for breast cancer; the surgery had been successful, and she was considered out of danger. A complication arose, however. She returned to her surgeon repeatedly, complaining of pain.

"I can't find anything wrong," he said.

"But I really am feeling this pain all the time," she insisted.

"As far as medicine is concerned," he replied, "your pain doesn't exist."

Feeling extremely frustrated, the woman was advised by a friend to go for an Ayurvedic consultation. On examination it was determined that she was a Kapha type, which ordinarily predicts very good health. But the traumas her body had been subjected to during her illness had led to a gross imbalance of Vata dosha. Her medical history showed that since her surgery she had complained repeatedly to her doctors, not just of pain but of not being able to sleep well. Her profile of Vata symptoms was very clear, particularly when you consider that any wound such as major surgery drastically aggravates Vata dosha.

It was explained to her that although doctors tend to look for gross physical causes behind every pain, there are countless patients like her who were responding to pain caused by imbalanced Vata. Although linked to the body, Vata is a separate, subtler part of the whole mind body system.

She was put on a program to balance her Vata—something that should be done for every postoperative patient—including a special diet, rest, and meditation. In short order her pain was reduced to tolerable limits, her insomnia cleared up, and her constant anxiety disappeared. A skeptic might contend that "phantom pain" was at work here, a mysterious phenomenon that is often seen in amputees. But the subjective experience of pain is all that really matters, not its name. Using the doshas to explore a new level of reality proves extremely helpful in making sense of otherwise inexplicable illness.

A good example is peptic ulcers. There is recent evidence that in the vast majority of cases, the presence of bacteria called *Helicobacter pylori* is associated with stomach ulcers. Eradicating this germ with antibiotics cures the ulcer in more than 90 percent of cases. Therefore, the current medical model considers stomach ulcers to be an infectious disease.

This would seem simple enough except for the fact that almost half of the world's population harbors *Helicobacter pylori* in their digestive tract, but only 10 to 20 percent develop peptic ulcer diseases. Therefore, we have to ask why most people with these bacteria do not get an ulcer. From an Ayurvedic perspective the answer is that individuals have different responses to challenges from the environment, based upon their doshas.

According to Ayurveda, the typical ulcer victim is a textbook case of Pitta imbalance. When you look up Pitta aggravation, you find the same constellation of symptoms that afflicts an ulcer patient.

Symptoms of Pitta Imbalance

Inflammation of digestive tract
Excess gastric juice
Anger, hostility, tension
Burning sensation in digestive tract
Excess acidity in body

This list reads like a guidebook to getting an ulcer, but it is actually a guide to what happens before the ulcer occurs. Since the doshas can be a little out of balance or a lot, a Pitta imbalance does not guarantee that a peptic ulcer is about to appear. However, in people who have strong Pitta natures, ulcers are a common complaint, possibly because the way Pitta people deal with stress leads to changes in their stomach acid secretion and weakness in their immune systems. Preventing Pitta imbalances in the first place, using Ayurvedic diet, exercise, meditation, and so forth may help maintain the healthy defenses necessary to avoid an ulcer.

Let's take note of a potentially sensitive point here. To participate in a disease is not to cause it. If you go out into the cold without your hat and coat, you may catch a cold. If that happens, your heedless actions played their part, even though a microbiologist would be right to assert that you did not *cause* your cold—a virus did. In Ayurveda, more responsibility is being put on your shoulders, on your ability to learn about your own dosha makeup. I am not saying, "When you get right down to it, you caused your cancer, your heart attack, your case of AIDS." But I do feel that you are not separate from these diseases; in fact, being an active participant is what saves us from being helpless victims.

In Ayurveda, we don't tend to talk much about germs, which are basically well understood in the West already. What is poorly understood are "host defenses." This is where knowing your own doshas really pays off. If you expose yourself directly to cold viruses, your chance of actually coming down with a cold is only about 1 in 8. Why? Because your inner state of balance is the deciding factor. Keeping your doshas healthy makes all the difference.

In the following pages you will find a comprehensive description of imbalance, dosha by dosha. Then, in chapter 5, we'll explore the Ayurvedic techniques for restoring balance in the most natural, comfortable way.

HOW THE DOSHAS GET UNBALANCED

The dosha that is most likely to go out of balance is the one that dominates your body type, meaning that Vatas should be careful about aggravating their Vata, Pittas their Pitta, and so on. If you are a two-dosha type, both doshas are possible candidates for causing problems. However, in everyone the most active dosha is always Vata. It leads to the majority of short-term problems, particularly if they are stress-related. (See chapter 5, "Restoring the Balance," for more about the role Vata plays as "king" of the doshas.)

The typical signs of dosha imbalance are given here, along with some of the most common conditions that cause them.

Vata Imbalance

By nature a Vata person is cheerful, enthusiastic, and resilient in the face of life's everyday challenges. If you are a Vata type and have retained these qualities, you are very likely in balance. It is undeniable, however, that Vatas do not generally enjoy the best health. In childhood or adolescence they begin to have various problems: unexplained aches and pains, occasional sleeplessness, or a pronounced tendency to be worried and nervous.

In time, if these early signs are not heeded, Vatas become the most common visitors to doctors' waiting rooms, accounting for the huge number of prescriptions written for sleeping pills, tranquilizers, and pain relievers. One would be justified in saying that the most common disorder in America is Vata aggravation. Not that American life is solely to blame; Ayurveda holds that Vata dosha causes twice the complaints as Pitta, and Pitta twice the number as Kapha. Typical Vata complaints of headache, backache, insomnia, menstrual cramps, and low-level anxiety or depression are considered symptoms of the "worried well" by many doctors. However, they are very real, stubborn problems that need to be addressed by bringing Vata back into balance.

Other scenes from life also present a picture of classic Vata imbalance. One is the picture of old age, a time when Vata increases in everyone. Aging badly can bring out the worst signs of Vata aggravation: the person shrivels into a bag of skin and bones; he no longer enjoys eating and has trouble digesting his food; his mind wanders and becomes forgetful; he spends long, lonely nights without being able to sleep. None of these things is caused by Vata; they are caused by Vata imbalance and therefore can be prevented.

Another picture is that of grief. People who have gone into deep mourning will become listless and apathetic, refuse to eat, and take no enjoyment from anything in life. It is as if the shock of death has deadened them, too. Since Vata controls the nervous system, this is in fact what has happened. Grief, a sudden shock, battle fatigue, or great fear exhausts Vata dosha, and it loses its ability to register perception. The first stage of the process is usually marked by weeping, restless behavior, shakiness, racing thoughts, and lack of sleep. If the stress is deep enough or protracted enough, however, the inevitable result is that Vata collapses, leading to total apathy and lack of response.

WHY DID IT HAPPEN?

If you start to feel sick and the cause is Vata imbalance, there is usually a precipitating cause that can be pointed out and corrected. Being born a Vata type or having a strong amount of Vata in your constitution is certainly a strong predisposing factor. On the other hand, it takes a pattern of behavior to actually throw this dosha out of balance. Among the most typical patterns to look for are:

- You have been under stress recently and reacted to it with anxiety.
- You have exhausted yourself physically or undergone a period of mental strain and overwork.
- You are in the advanced stages of alcohol or drug addiction, or you chain-smoke.
- There has been a sudden change in your life, or the seasons are changing.
- Your diet includes a great deal of cold, raw, or dry foods, including iced beverages; or you eat a great many bitter, spicy, or astringent foods. (Bitter and astringent tastes show up primarily in salads, beans, potatoes, and leafy green vegetables.)
- You have been on a stringent diet or habitually skip meals. Going on an empty stomach and ignoring the body's hunger signals increases Vata.
- You have gone without sleep or slept poorly for more than a few days.

- You have taken a trip recently.
- You have suffered emotionally from grief, fear, or unexpected shock.
- The weather is cold, dry, and windy (autumn/winter).

In clinical practice, an Ayurvedic doctor would diagnose Vata imbalance if he found strong evidence of the following kind:

MENTAL INDICATIONS

Worry, anxiety	Loss of mental focus
Overactive mind	Short attention span
Impatience	Depression, psychosis

BEHAVIORAL INDICATIONS

Insomnia	Restlessness
Fatigue	Low appetite
Inability to relax	Impulsiveness

PHYSICAL INDICATIONS

Constipation	Irritable bowel syndrome
Dry or rough skin	Chapped skin, lips
Low stamina, loss of energy	Intolerance to cold and wind
Intestinal gas, flatulence	Aching or arthritic joints
High blood pressure	Weight loss, emaciated tissues
Lower back pain	Acute pain (especially nerve
Menstrual cramps	pain)
Muscle spasms, seizures	

It is important to remember that any dosha can cause any symptom—these are just the most common signs of a Vata imbalance. Also, Vata can mimic the other two doshas, so it often comes under suspicion even when its typical symptoms are not present.

Pitta Imbalance

Pitta people are in balance when their built-in intensity and drive are not overwhelming; to be sweet-natured and joyous are also innate Pitta qualities. If you are a Pitta type and these are still present, you are likely to be in balance. The physical health of Pitta types is generally good. Its foundation is strong digestion, which Ayurveda considers the key to building healthy tissues and preserving a strong immune status.

Life's middle years, from adolescence until the end of middle age, are the time when everyone's Pitta increases. A teenager suffering from acne or from feeling too hot at night is exhibiting Pitta imbalance. Another very common picture of aggravated Pitta is the man in his thirties or forties who wakes up to find that his hair is thinning at an alarming rate or turning prematurely gray, who suddenly needs eyeglasses, or who has developed heartburn or early heart disease.

Some of these are predisposed conditions, but Pittas also tend to go out of balance by pushing themselves to extremes. On the assumption that they can eat anything, they abuse their strong digestion by overeating or forgetting about nutrition. Instead of being natural high achievers, they can become driving, impatient, demanding, and tense. Pitta dosha controls the intellect and endows Pitta types with a sense of orderliness. Out of balance, they become fixated on order and annoyingly perfectionist. Pittas don't display such traits until they go seriously out of balance, and then it is not surprising that they also become prey to heartburn, ulcers, heart disease, and other stress-related problems.

Pitta dosha is slower to go out of balance than Vata and is said to cause about half the problems that Vata does. When it does go out, Pitta is frequently being dragged along by an earlier imbalance of Vata. This one-two combination accounts for undercurrents of anxiety that angry, critical people are trying desperately to hide; aggravated Vata also promotes the high blood pressure that doctors often see among their Type A heart patients.

WHY DID IT HAPPEN?

If you start to feel sick and the cause is Pitta imbalance, the fault is not that you were born a Pitta type or with strong Pitta in your makeup. By nature Pitta is inclined to moderation, and you have to build up a history of excessive stress, overwork, or sheer thoughtlessness to break down this instinct. If you think aggravated Pitta is at work, look for the following causes and try to correct them:

- You have been under stress and have reacted to it with suppressed anger, frustration, and resentment.
- You place excessive demands on yourself and others, live under constant pressure from deadlines, and cannot bear to waste time.
- You have eaten too much hot, spicy food, oily food, or fried food recently; you use a great deal of salt. Your diet contains a large amount of sour or fermented foods: cheese, vinegar, sour cream, or alcoholic beverages.
- You have been exposed to impure food and water.
- The weather is hot and humid (typical summer weather).
- You have been heat-fatigued or badly sunburned.

In his medical practice, an Ayurvedic doctor identifies Pitta imbalance with the following patterns of symptoms:

MENTAL INDICATIONS

Anger, hostility

Self-criticism

Irritability, impatience

Resentment

BEHAVIORAL INDICATIONS

Outbursts of temper

Argumentative stance

Tyrannical behavior

Criticism of others

Intolerance of delays

PHYSICAL INDICATIONS

Skin inflammations, boils, rashes

Acne

Excessive hunger or thirst

Bad breath

Hot flashes

Heartburn, acid stomach

Ulcers

Sour body odors

Rectal burning, hemorrhoids

Patchy, florid complexion

Intolerance to heat

Bloodshot eyes

Sunburn, sunstroke

Pronounced yellowing of feces and urine

It is important to remember that any dosha can cause any symptom—these are just the most common signs of a Pitta imbalance.

Kapha Imbalance

Kapha is the slowest and steadiest of the doshas, which makes it reluctant to go out of balance. From childhood on,

Kapha types are serene, calm, affectionate, and forgiving. If you are a Kapha type and these qualities are still intact, you are very likely in balance. Disorders related to Kapha generally take a long time to develop. Without much effort, therefore, Kapha people can expect to remain strong, healthy, and content to a ripe old age.

Infancy and childhood are Kapha times of life, when this dosha increases in everyone. Kapha is identified with growth and the production of a strong, healthy body. To imagine what Kapha is like out of balance, think of a 6-year-old with a chronic sore throat and runny nose who catches one cold after another. Otherwise healthy Kaphas may retain this weakness for life, frequently suffering from blocked sinuses or a pronounced susceptibility to colds and flu when the weather turns chilly and damp.

Allergies might also be present, along with a strong desire to oversleep. Kapha types generally like to stay in bed and are slow starters, but when they are out of balance, they become so sluggish in the morning that they worry about serious illness when the real problem in most cases is too much Kapha.

In later years, the picture of Kapha imbalance becomes the jolly fat man, an insecure person who cannot control his overweight or his distress about it. Being clinging and possessive is also a mark of disturbed Kapha, where the natural tendency to mother and care for others has been pushed to an extreme. If this dosha becomes seriously imbalanced, the person can become very quiet, withdrawn, and hopeless; the Kapha tendency to value the status quo then turns into a rigid inability to accept change. Physically, the jolly fat man can come to a pathetic end, suffering from gross hypertension, labored breathing, bloating from excess bodily fluids, and congestive heart failure.

Kaphas do not go to the doctor very often, because they are able to tolerate high levels of pain and are also used to being extremely healthy. When they do seek medical attention, it is either for overweight, which can set in as early as childhood and continue for life, or various lung and sinus problems— sinus headaches, chronic sinusitis, hay fever, asthma, chest congestion.

Doctors have found that only a tiny percentage of people who think they have food allergies test positive when given patch tests; what is generally wrong is a digestive imbalance, with Kapha a prime suspect. Excess mucus is being pro- duced by wheat bread or pasta, milk, butter, cheese, or sugar, all of which aggravate this dosha. Diabetes, perhaps the most dangerous Kapha disorder, is among the most unlikely to be cured. However, diabetics can lead much more com- fortable and stable lives if they follow the proper body-type program.

Why Did It Happen?

If you start to feel sick and the cause is Kapha imbalance, usually you will either have a passing cold or flu, or else there is a pattern of illness you detected early on in your life— allergies, asthma, obesity, and so on. In either case, the follow- ing influences are likely to be present, either causing or aggravating your condition:

- A serious Kapha problem, such as diabetes, allergies, or obesity, runs in your family.
- You have gained a lot of weight and feel depressed about it.

- Your diet contains large amounts of sugar, salt, fatty or fried foods, heavy foods, dairy products (especially cheese, milk, and ice cream).
- You have been under stress and react to it by withdrawing, feeling insecure and unwanted.
- You place excessive emphasis on possessing, storing, and saving things.
- You act dependent or overprotective in relationships.
- You have been sleeping late more than a few days in a row.
- The weather is cold and damp or snowy (typical winter and spring weather).

In medical practice, an Ayurvedic physician diagnoses Kapha imbalance by looking for the following symptoms:

MENTAL INDICATIONS

Dullness, mental inertia	Stupor, depression
Lassitude	Overattachment

BEHAVIORAL INDICATIONS

Procrastination	Balkiness
Inability to accept change	Slow movements
Greed	Possessiveness
Oversleeping, drowsiness	

PHYSICAL INDICATIONS

Intolerance of cold and damp	Heaviness in limbs
Sinus congestion, runny nose	Frequent colds
Fluid retention in tissues, bloating	Weight gain
	Allergies, asthma

Chest congestion	Phlegmy cough, sore throat
Skin pallor	
Loose or aching joints	Cysts and other growths
High cholesterol	Diabetes

It is important to remember that any dosha can cause any symptom—these are just the most common signs of a Kapha imbalance.

CHAPTER 5

RESTORING THE BALANCE

$\mathbf{M}$ichelangelo's genius as a sculptor lay in his ability to see a finished statue inside a rough block of marble. His challenge was not to make a sculpture but to release the one that was already there, imprisoned in the stone. Essentially that is what you do when you bring yourself back into balance. You are not creating a new you; you are releasing a hidden you. The process is one of self-discovery.

The hidden you that wants to emerge is in perfect balance. Finding it is not a rote affair—every person achieves balance in his or her personal way. Most people have no idea who they really are—or at best a very limited idea—because they have no way to see their true nature. It is hidden from them by their imbalances, like a lake bottom hidden by muddy water. Like hunger and thirst, the instinct for balance is built into the human body. In the practice of Ayurveda we try to bring people back into balance and at the same time let their true nature shine through. The two processes are really the same, as the following case study will show.

❖

By his own estimate, Norman, a writer in his early sixties, has not had a good night's sleep in thirty years. Norman's insomnia is the classic Vata kind: as soon as he gets into bed, his mind finds a dozen things to worry about, and a hundred impressions from the day whirl in his head. He cannot keep his attention off them, or off the ticking clock, the dripping faucet, and the noises coming in from the street. He tosses restlessly all night without feeling that he has slept for more than a half-hour at a stretch.

By the time he comes to see us, he is very discouraged, having tried a long string of sleep remedies, from whiskey nightcaps to barbiturates, none of which worked for long. Over time, he has resigned himself to his fate, but only superficially—actually, Norman dreads bedtime and delays it every night as long as he can. He keeps magazines piled by his side to read whenever he wakes up. If he is too restless to read, he paces the floor, goes to the bathroom, eats a midnight snack, or calls his insomniac friends for long night-owl chats.

"It's all because I'm Vata, isn't it?" he mourns, having learned about the prakruti system through reading about Ayurveda and taking a prakruti test.

"There's certainly Vata imbalance here," he is told, "but that doesn't make you a Vata type." He looks surprised. A thorough examination discloses that he is mainly Pitta, with a strong Vata component. Even so, it is not his Vata that made him insomniac but a history of throwing Vata dosha out of balance, largely by the constant use of his mind: Norman worked on his writing at all hours of the day and night and had never seriously considered being completely regular in his habits. If he had, his Vata aggravation might not have grown so bad over the years.

To make him see the healthier person inside himself, we began to explain how balance works and how temporary imbalances become permanent.

A HUNDRED THERMOSTATS

Every function in the body has a home base it wants to return to, just as a thermostat has its fixed set point. In fact, body temperature operates very much like a thermostat. You can raise it by running half a mile or sitting inside a sauna, but after you stop, your temperature will return to 98.6 degrees F. That is home base for your body's thermostat, established by natural laws over the course of evolution. These laws are flexible, so you can temporarily depart from the normal setting of 98.6, but if you depart too far or too long, there will be unpleasant repercussions.

One of the main reasons why human physiology is so complex is that hundreds of thermostats have been installed inside us, each obeying its own special set of natural laws—we have not just one single balance point but many. Their coordination is quite miraculous. You would think that the bloodstream, for example, would be a stew of biochemicals, considering the bewildering number of hormones, nutrients, and diverse messenger molecules that float through it. In fact, the bloodstream is so exactly balanced that all these molecules go where they are needed with exquisitely precise timing and in exact measure.

Similarly, the brain is capable of keeping track of all our overlapping thermostats without confusion. One tiny portion of gray matter in the fore-brain, called the hypothalamus, weighing roughly one-sixth of an ounce, is responsible for balancing an amazing number of diverse functions, including fat and carbohydrate metabolism, sleeping and waking, appetite, thirst, digestive secretions, levels of fluids, growth, body temperature—in short, everything that goes on automatically inside the body. Whatever you do not have to think about is being looked after by your hypothalamus (sometimes called "the brain's brain").

What this shows is that balance is a function of intelligence. We are not really a collection of thermostats, because a thermostat cannot set itself: we can. The original setting that you were born with is your prakruti, or given nature. It serves as a guide, but you can manipulate it. Let's say that someone was born with a Pitta-Vata setting, as Norman was. We can illustrate this prakruti with a simple diagram:

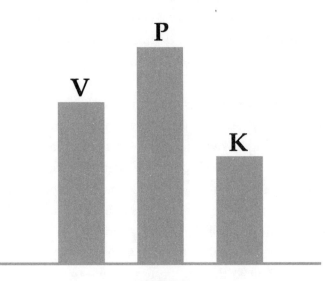

PRAKRUTI

At birth, this set point determines the ideal balance for the three doshas during the person's whole lifetime. All of the hundreds of thermostats in the body obey this master setting, just as they obey your hypothalamus. But you can talk to your doshas much more easily than you can to your hypothalamus. Vata predictably goes up when any aggravating influence, such as cold weather, dry or moving air, fear, the taste of spicy food, and staying up too late at night, touches it. These influences are the words that say "more Vata" to the body. (Pitta and Kapha have their own catalysts.)

The baby who came into this world as a Pitta-Vata may grow up to look like a very different adult:

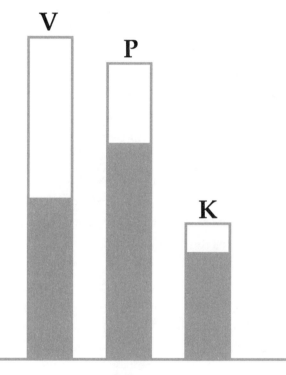

VIKRUTI

Now it appears that he is a Vata-Pitta, because the doshas have been moved to new positions by the everyday influences of life, including food, exercise, sleep, and emotions. Everything you think, say, do, see, feel, smell, or taste moves your doshas, either a little or a lot. They are meant to bounce back after traveling to a new position, following their instinct for balance. In this case, as in Norman's, something went wrong.

The shaded zone is now topped by a blank area, standing for the imbalances that have accumulated over time. They are called *vikruti* in Ayurveda, a word that means "deviating from nature." The two terms prakruti and vikruti are thus opposites, one referring to what is natural for a person, the other to what is not. You cannot push your doshas into a configuration that is better than the one you were born with; you will only create distance between yourself and nature. Skip a meal and you add a little to your vikruti; go without sleep for a night and you add a little more. Wrong food, bad sleeping habits, negative emotions, and physical or mental strain all make life a little bit more unnatural, until eventually you find yourself in the most unnatural of all conditions, a full-blown disease.

At the same time, your self-image will also change—in place of positive reactions, you will start to display more negative ones. Vikruti makes you more sensitive to stresses of all kinds. It tarnishes the finer emotions. How many of us still feel the innocent capacity to love and trust that a baby is born with? We crowd our cells with all the experiences of rejection, disappointment, and doubt that litter everyone's past. You may now think of yourself as a born worrier or a lifelong insomniac, pessimist, or a grouch, forgetting that it took years to become that way.

In Norman's vikruti, Vata dosha is the one that is most severely aggravated. This is not surprising, since Vata is the easiest dosha to perturb. Vata dislikes such things as loud noise, crowds, and physical discomfort, so when you get on a packed commuter train, your body will register the experience as stress. The more you ride, the more Vata will be aggravated. In time, the very idea of commuting to work arouses unpleasant reactions: you will adapt to them, but you will never thrive. In this way, the doshas guide us toward right habits and away from wrong ones.

"Right" simply means close to nature. It is right to give Vata a period of absolute peace and quiet every day; this allows it to find its balance point. It is wrong to abuse Vata with loud noise and overcrowding, because that throws it further out of balance. "Everyone has to earn a living," you may think, getting on the same commuter train tomorrow and again the day after. Nothing will make Vata enjoy the experience, though. This is one of the most fortunate things in the world, for your only hope of returning to perfect balance is the instinct every dosha has to resist wrong treatment and return to home base.

Norman found it very easy to recognize his situation in all of this. "Turning into an unnatural Vata-Pitta is very common in our society," he was informed, "given how much aggravation surrounds us in the environment."

"But vikruti is a mask, an illusion built out of stress. Underneath is that original ideal setting, the unique combination of Vata, Pitta, and Kapha that is the real you. If it can be recovered, your Vata symptoms will disappear. The beauty of Ayurveda is that it makes people healthy by returning them to their best selves."

The next step was to give Norman a new routine to follow, one that would soothe his disturbed doshas. We gave him a list of things that bring aggravated Vata back into balance—the process called "pacifying a dosha." (At the end of this chapter you will find general recommendations for pacifying the three doshas; details will be elaborated as we go deeper into the practice of Ayurveda.) First on the list was faithful regularity to the same daily habits. In Norman's case, he quickly formulated a nighttime ritual.

"An hour before bedtime I take a warm bath—a little cooler in the summer. Then I lightly massage my forehead, temples, and feet with sesame oil for five minutes and drink a glass of warm milk with a *rasayana* mixed in." (Rasayanas are herbal compounds, of which Ayurveda has hundreds; Norman finds that the most general rasayana, Biochavan, is very effective, but there are specific Ayurvedic herbs that can also be substituted.)

"Next I sit quietly and read for twenty minutes. For me, the most relaxing reading is poetry or inspirational literature. Finally, I turn off the light and listen to soothing music until I feel drowsy, and then I immediately get into bed.

"I have followed this routine faithfully for four months, and without fail I fall asleep without difficulty and sleep at least six hours straight, which is enough for me to feel refreshed the next day."

All in all, a very happy outcome for a problem that millions of people suffer from without relief, despite the fact that an estimated one out of five Americans takes sleeping pills on a regular basis. This is not just an insomnia cure, either, since Norman enjoys the other benefits of getting into balance. He no longer complains of frequent colds or minor aches and pains. He has lost the worry and dissatisfaction that had become part of his makeup. He looks fresher overall, and life looks fresher through his eyes.

SIX STAGES OF DISEASE

Putting patients back in touch with their own nature has been the aim of medicine for thousands of years—it is not unique to Ayurveda. In the West, however, we have been spellbound by scientific medicine, with its strictly physical explanation for disease. Now Western medicine is conceding that illness can originate in either the body or the mind. With the advent of mind body medicine, it is no longer clear that these two can even be separated. A sudden mental shock, such as the death of a spouse, can create havoc in the body, crippling the immune system and opening the way for illness, which helps account for a much higher death rate among recent widows than among the general population. It suggests a rationale for why lonely women who lack the opportunity to give emotional support to others tend to have higher rates of breast cancer.

This shift toward mind body explanations has had both its good and bad sides. For example, we used to say that pneumonia begins when pneumococcus bacteria invade the lungs and start to multiply there uncontrollably. In mind body medicine, any explanation has its roots in an earlier stage, in the moment when the immune system was weakened by a negative mental influence. This is a broader explanation than the purely physical one, but, unfortunately, it is also quite vague. The interaction of the mind and the immune system is so fluid that doctors cannot actually pinpoint the critical moment when negative thoughts compromise the body's white cells.

In Ayurveda, we are able to be much more precise. According to the ancient texts, the disease process has six distinct phases or steps. The first three are invisible and can be tied in to either the body or the mind; the last three carry overt symptoms that can be detected by both the patient and his doctor. Each stage represents a loss of balance, but its appearance changes as the process continues:

1. Accumulation—the process begins with the buildup of one or more doshas.
2. Aggravation—the excess dosha accumulates to the point that it starts to spread outside its normal boundaries.
3. Dissemination—the dosha moves throughout the body.
4. Localization—the wandering dosha settles somewhere it does not belong.
5. Manifestation—physical symptoms arise at the point where the dosha has localized.
6. Disruption—a full-blown disease erupts.

To illustrate these steps, let's say that excess Pitta has accumulated, perhaps because you are a Pitta type who finds himself under heavy stress or just suffering through the discomfort of a very hot summer. Once there is enough excess Pitta accumulated, it starts to move around the body, leaving the places where it is supposed to remain. In short order it finds a place where *ama* (toxic residue) is present; it now gets "stuck" to the ama.

This event concludes the first three stages of disease. At this point, a Western doctor would not yet have a diagnosis, because no textbook disorder is present, but it is certain from the Ayurvedic standpoint that the body is no longer perfectly healthy. If you are very aware of your body, you can sense the initial onset of a dosha imbalance. Everyone recognizes the subtle changes that indicate a cold or flu is on the way. For many other diseases, feeling "out of sorts" registers as a vague discomfort that cannot be localized or identified. It usually baffles the doctor, who tries to find overt symptoms but runs up against a fuzzy constellation of aches, pains, muscle weakness, low-grade fever, or simply lingering fatigue. This sort of vague premonition in the body holds true even for a sudden heart attack or stroke, which is rarely sudden at all. The victim is usually given warnings in advance by his doshas but doesn't heed them.

Once a dosha gets stuck somewhere, it generally ushers in the fourth stage, when the first distinct symptoms of sickness begin to appear. If the Pitta has lodged in the skin, you may feel a little itching or inflammation. If it is in the stomach, you may feel heartburn or upset stomach. (We are not blaming just Pitta for disease symptoms. Any dosha can lodge anywhere. If excess Vata has lodged in a joint, one of the most likely places for it since joints readily pick up ama, you might feel a twinge of arthritis.) Except for such vague signs, there is still no indication that a serious disease might be in the offing.

Because Ayurveda works at such a subtle level of our bodies, symptoms can be relieved that are often quite mysterious by Western standards, including unexplainable pain, anxiety, depression, fatigue, and so on. Western medicine tends to say that these are psychosomatic problems, that is, that they originate in the patient's head. In truth, they originate at the early stages of dosha imbalance. It is easy to manage them while they are still in stages 1, 2, or 3, when diet, herbs, exercise, daily routine, and a special purification technique for the body called panchakarma (to be discussed shortly) can all be effectively employed.

Once we are dealing with full-blown illness, the damage to bodily tissues often goes far beyond what these treatments alone can undo. Then we must progress to more advanced Ayurvedic therapies, or call in Western medicine, which has been formulated to deal with acute conditions of all sorts.

How do you know when stage 4—the first onset of symptoms—is about to commence? For most adults over 40, there is no need to look too far, since we experience vague aches and pains with distressing frequency. Bodies subjected to dietary, behavioral, and emotional imbalance over the years will always collect ama, and ama by its nature will catch a wandering dosha. There is no cause for alarm, however. What your body is telling you at stage 4 is not that you are in grave danger but that you need to purify your tissues of excess doshas. Once you do, Vata, Pitta, and Kapha will regain their natural balance. The basic approach of "talking" to the doshas via simple changes in diet and daily routine can bring dramatic results, even in cases of serious illness.

HOW TO BALANCE YOUR DOSHAS

In the following pages, I give the general guidelines for bringing Vata, Pitta, and Kapha back into balance. There are four broad areas of everyday life that can be used to promote balance:

Diet   Exercise   Daily routine   Seasonal routine

I devote separate sections to each of these later, in part III; for now, they will be discussed in more general terms to give you a basic understanding of how you can affect your doshas—a primer on living from your quantum mechanical body.

One important caution: The points given here are intended *for prevention only*. They are not suitable for treating diseases or as a substitute for a doctor's care. If you have any symptoms of illness, restoring your dosha balance is vital, but it is not the whole story. You need a complete examination by a trained physician, who will guide you in a complete medical regime suited to your specific situation.

For all of us in good health, however, the following information is invaluable and unique. The points were collected over five years of consulting the ancient Ayurvedic texts, collecting the wisdom of living Ayurvedic authorities in India, and using our own experience with thousands of patients in the United States at the Chopra Center.

Please be flexible about the advice being offered here. These are not rigid rules to be agonized over. You can waste a lifetime running after the goal of balance and never attain it, because the doshas shift by the hour, by the day, by the minute. And yet balance is the easiest thing of all. Nature has already endowed your body with the proper instincts for it; our principles only help to uncover and sharpen those instincts.

For most people, the worst temptation is diet. Each of us is probably a little fanatical about foods we think must be good or bad for us. Because Ayurveda has so much to say about food, it can be easily used to support an obsession with diet. But if you see it in the proper light, all this new information is just a way to wake up your body. Ayurveda doesn't dictate that one food is "right" and another "wrong." Instead, you discover right and wrong by listening to your doshas.

So don't get caught up in the details of whether your food is too hot or too cold, too heavy or too light, too oily or too dry. Every time a dosha moves, some specific food could be called upon to keep the body from losing balance. But if we approach balance this way, the process rapidly degenerates into fanaticism. This is not the way of self-knowledge. Every day is a conversation between you and your body; the following suggestions indicate the kind of talk your body type generally likes to hear.

THE BALANCED LIFE—GENERAL POINTS

Balancing Vata

- Regular habits
- Quiet
- Attention to fluids
- Decreased sensitivity to stress
- Ample rest
- Warmth
- Steady supply of nourishment
- Sesame oil massage (*abhyanga*)

Because Vata is "king" of the doshas, balancing it is a prime requirement for everyone; when Vata is brought into line, it will bring Pitta and Kapha with it.

The key to balancing Vata dosha is regularity. Vata is so sensitive and quick to change that it easily falls prey to overstimulation. Vata people thrive on variety, but when things change too much, their excitement turns to exhaustion. That is why so many Vatas feel frazzled and nervous. The source of their restlessness is that Vata dosha is no longer setting the proper rhythms in their bodies. Instead of eating, sleeping, and exercising regularly, out-of-balance Vatas grab food when they can, skip meals, exercise by fits and starts, and go to bed at odd hours.

Such a life is bad for all the doshas, but it is worse for Vata. Many Vata types cling to it. Sadly, they have conditioned themselves to feel that a haphazard life is the same as a stimulating one. The remedy is to begin to cultivate balanced habits, paying a little more attention to regularity every day.

If you show signs of Vata imbalance, these pointers will help you reshape your daily routine to make it more congenial to Vata dosha:

- Get plenty of rest—this is all-important for any Vata problem. When you feel that you are pushing yourself or overdoing any activity (including mental activity), stop and rest for five minutes. Getting adequate sleep every night is also of utmost importance; you shouldn't resign yourself to insomnia, even though you may have had it for years. The best rest, aside from sleep, is the deep relaxation provided by meditation. At the Chopra Center we offer every patient the opportunity to learn Primordial Sound Meditation (PSM) in order to experience profound relaxation. The dosha to benefit most is Vata, which emerges thoroughly settled and refreshed after only a few minutes of meditation.

There is a much deeper benefit to be gained as well. Meditation helps to integrate the mind body link. This in turn allows every natural cycle in the body to come full circle, to progress smoothly through a beginning, middle, and end. When Vatas find that fulfillment is a permanent state within themselves, not a rare flower to be chased after, they take a huge step forward in finding out who they really are.

- Stay warm—being a cold dosha, Vata benefits from heat; Vata is also dry, so be sure that the air in your room has enough humidity. It is advisable to avoid drafts, too, since Vata is extremely sensitive to moving air.

- Eat a Vata-pacifying diet (see page 262). It is also important for you to eat regularly, since Vata dosha is aggravated by an empty stomach. Vata types waste away quickly when they feel sick or stop eating regularly. They need to be nourished throughout the day, even though their appetites will ordinarily be variable. Make sure you sit down to three meals a day, including a warm, nourishing breakfast of substantial foods, such as hot cereal. Taking a little fresh ginger helps to stimulate the appetite before the meal and aids digestion.

- Drink lots of *warm* fluids during the day to prevent dehydration. Vata herb tea, available by mail order, is the best choice; you can drink up to four cups a day. Fresh ginger-root tea, prepared by placing a teaspoon of fresh grated ginger into a pint thermos bottle and filling it with hot water, is also Vata pacifying. Avoid very cold food and drinks.

- Massage your body with sesame oil in the morning. This Ayurvedic routine is called *abhyanga* (see page 250 for details).
- Take a long, warm bath or shower in the morning before you meditate. Moist heat is good for Vata aches and pains.
- Avoid mental strain and overstimulating yourself. Loud music, violent movies, and long hours of TV, particularly in the evening, are all potent aggravators of Vata.
- Make your surroundings light and bright. Vata responds well to sunlight and cheerful colors. If you are sick, sitting before a closed window in the sun is a good idea. Resist the urge to go outdoors for any length of time until you are well, however. See people who make you cheerful, read humorous books, watch light, humorous entertainment. Anything that brings out Vata's natural enthusiasm and reduces worry will be very helpful.
- Do not drink alcohol while you are trying to balance Vata, which resents stimulants of any kind, including coffee, tea, and nicotine. All of these have to be handled with care by anyone sensitive to Vata imbalances. The ideal is to give them up altogether.
- Vatas often have dry nasal passages in winter, which contributes to the frequency of catching colds. To offset this, place a drop of sesame oil on the tip of your finger and rub it gently inside one nostril; repeat with the other nostril. Now pinch your nose and start to inhale, then rapidly release and pinch again to draw sesame oil into the nasal cavities—do not strain, however, or try to unblock the sinuses.

  This treatment is particularly soothing in dry, cold weather—many Vata types notice that their resistance to colds and flu is helped considerably—but it also tones the sinuses in general and can be used by everyone, not just Vatas. The treatment can be repeated up to twelve times a day. (If your sinuses are blocked, however, you should not overdo this treatment; oil aggravates Kapha dosha, which is often behind chronic sinusitis.)

Balancing Pitta

- Moderation
- Coolness
- Attention to leisure
- Exposure to natural beauty
- Balance of rest and activity
- Decreased stimulants

The key to balancing Pitta is moderation, making sure that you do not push yourself too hard. Of all the body types, Pitta is gifted with the most innate drive, aggression, and energy. Pittas are people who attack life head-on and relish challenges, the more difficult the better. But this inner drive is often the source of their undoing. Pitta gives you a fiery energy; if you abuse it, it will burn you up. The workaholics of this world are generally out-of-balance Pittas, especially if their emotional undertone is angry and compulsive.

Pitta types have to consciously pull themselves back when they see certain danger signs, the most obvious being loss of sweetness in their emotions and loss of moderation in their appetites. There is also a built-in love of beauty that is important in the Pitta nature. In all the points listed below, the main theme for Pitta is "the good life is the one that follows a golden mean."

If you show signs of Pitta imbalance, the following pointers will help balance your daily routine and make it more congenial to Pitta dosha:

- Take time to wind down from activity—alternating rest and activity is the basic rhythm of life. Because they have so much capacity for activity, Pittas tend to ignore the other side of the cycle. You need to find an island of calm at the end of your workday. Eat a quiet dinner, turn off your telephone in the evening, and resolutely avoid the temptation to bring your work home. For all of us, the island of calm is really inside ourselves. Out-of-balance Pittas frequently lose sight of this.

- Meditation is very useful for regaining inner calm and equilibrium. It also allows you to remember that rest is the source of dynamic activity. The secret of great runners is not after all in their stride; it lies in the power they gather inside themselves on the starting block, before they take the first step. When Pittas discover that the greatest personal power is achieved without aggression, they take a huge step toward finding out who they really are.

- Coolness in any form helps to counteract overactive Pitta. Keep your bedroom just below 70 degrees when you sleep and don't linger in a hot bath too long; too much moist heat can make you feel dizzy or nauseated when Pitta is out of balance. If you feel overheated at any time, put a cool compress on your forehead and the back of your neck instead of drinking too much cold water. (Ice water, which puts out the digestive fire, is frowned on in Ayurveda.) Cool, sweet beverages that are not too sour are also good (apple juice, grape juice, club soda). Be sure to drink plenty of fluids in hot weather or if you feel sick; Pittas tend to perspire more and lose a lot of water under these conditions. A special Pitta-pacifying herb tea can be mail-ordered; you can drink up to four cups a day.

- Eat a Pitta-pacifying diet. It's important not to overeat, which Pittas tend to do if they push their excellent digestion too hard. At the same time, you don't want to feel uncomfortably hungry—Pittas suffer if they have to skip meals. Rather than going to extremes, eat moderate meals at regular hours three times a day. If your digestion is rocky, warm milk flavored with sugar and cardamom will help bring Pitta back into balance. If you always find yourself with a roaring appetite and excessive thirst, you need to moderate your digestion, which a Pitta-pacifying diet will help do (see page 270).

- If you find that you have a runaway appetite, do not try to force yourself to eat less. Instead, take gradually smaller meals, starting with about three-quarters of what you normally eat. Consume this amount for a day or two, then cut back to half of your normal consumption. Now you should be at a comfortable level of intake. Continue with this amount unless you feel uncomfortably hungry, in which case you should go back to the first reduction. If you are eating approximately two handfuls of food at each meal, you have reached the Ayurvedic ideal. (This regime originally comes from Charaka, the greatest ancient authority on Ayurveda.) The taste of bitter food curbs the appetite more than any other, so try drinking tonic water before a meal or eating a salad of bitter greens, such as chicory, endive, radicchio, and romaine lettuce.

- Avoid artificial stimulants, all of which raise Pitta. Alcohol in any form is like throwing kerosene on the Pitta fire (even fermented yeast in bread is not considered good for balancing Pitta). You do not need to stoke your digestive furnace with the empty calories in alcohol. The drawback of the caffeine in coffee and tea is that it puts an edge on your energy, while you need to smooth your edges.

- Traditionally, Ayurveda considers laxative treatment (*virechana*) the best way to reduce excess Pitta. This is because emptying the intestines for a brief time cools the "digestive fire." You can try taking one tablespoon of castor oil before bedtime once every four to six weeks (but not more often). Typically, the laxative will wake you up to go to the bathroom two or three times during the night; drink a glass of warm water after each elimination to avoid dehydration. The next day, when the body will feel lazy and relaxed, eat very little, taking perhaps a few glasses of fruit juice. If you eat solid food, avoid anything heavy, fatty, cold, or oily. Get plenty of rest. *However, do not take any laxatives if you have intestinal pain, bleeding, or a history of digestive complaints.*

- Be attentive to taking in only pure food, water, and air, since Pitta is especially sensitive to impurities of any kind. Food additives, even if judged harmless on the large scale, can create metabolic imbalances, however small, that interfere with your goal of achieving perfect balance.

- Avoid strenuous physical exertion or overheating yourself outdoors. Pittas are easily heat fatigued. Their pale skins, being intolerant of too much sun, will usually tell them when to go inside. Ayurveda recommends taking it very easy in the summer. Start with ten minutes in the direct sun and gradually work up to a half-hour, making sure to wear a protective sunscreen lotion. Morning and late afternoon are better times for you to be outside than high noon.

- Enjoy nature's beauty as often as possible—traditionally, Ayurveda recommends that Pitta types look at a sunset, watch the full moon, and walk beside lakes and running water. These are all appreciated by Pitta dosha. In general, Pitta people find a beautiful setting very conducive to winding down; it occupies their attention as sitting on the porch never could. Avoid reading books or watching shows that are violent, shocking, or controversial—all three influences strongly aggravate Pitta. Set aside some time every day for leisure that is uplifting, humorous, and entertaining—such influences help soften Pitta's edge. They also divert your tendency to become too wrapped up in your well-defined goals. Pittas already know how to be serious; they need the tonic of laughter more than any other type. In many ways, it is the best medicine for aggravated Pitta that nature has devised.

Balancing Kapha

- Stimulation
- Regular exercise
- Weight control
- Variety of experiences
- Warmth, dryness
- Reduced sweetness

The key to balancing Kapha is stimulation. By nature, Kapha dosha is steady and slow; this leads to dependability and strength. But out-of-balance Kaphas cling to the status quo too tightly; they need the stimulation of new sights and sounds, new people and events. The same is true physically. Without activity, Kaphas can become lethargic and dull. This is directly linked to their slow digestion. As we've seen, when food is not digested completely (or if it is too heavy, oily, or indigestible to begin with), toxic residues called ama can clog up the system and eventually lead to disease. Kapha types are particularly prone to this problem and need to make sure they keep their inner fire going through regular exercise and a varied diet.

Kapha people move in and out of balance slowly, so it is good to be steady about keeping this dosha in balance. Aggravate Vata today and you will likely feel the effects tomorrow. But you can eat Kapha-aggravating foods all winter and not realize your mistake until spring comes and the accumulated dosha "melts down," giving you a typical spring cold or sinus congestion. If you look at the list of the twenty-five gunas (see page 69), you will notice that Vata and Kapha do not share any qualities except coldness. As a result, Kapha people tend to need exactly the opposite of what Vatas need. This is why the Kapha strategy of stimulation is the opposite of the Vata rule of rest. Vatas are like rabbits, Kaphas like elephants.

If you show signs of Kapha imbalance, the following pointers will help make your daily routine more congenial to your dominant dosha.

- Seek variety in life. Kaphas need to make a conscious effort to seek new experiences. They cherish hearth and home, which averts the danger of running themselves ragged. But there is a definite tendency to stagnate, leading to depression, the bane of many unbalanced Kaphas. As with the other doshas, meditation is very useful here; it allows Kaphas to discover the underlying alertness in their nature.

  What makes life truly stimulating is not external variety but the spark of alertness inside us. Nature designed us to take a lively interest in fresh ideas, new faces, and productive innovation. (Man is the only creature, it is said, who will cross an ocean just to see what other men there look like.) With a little exposure to meditation, Kaphas who were content to watch the parade go by decide that what they really want is to join it. Kaphas are tempted to be possessive about life, to store and save everything that comes their way, whether it is money, energy, status, or love. When they discover that they can let go and use their solid strength as the fuel for change, they take a huge step forward in their personal evolution.

A Kapha's considerable capacity for loving and being loved then becomes twice as strong.

- Eat a Kapha-pacifying diet—it is important not to overeat if you are a Kapha type, because the tendency to become overweight is definitely present. Hot ginger tea taken at meals helps sharpen dulled taste buds; it also makes slow digestion more efficient, as does a teaspoon of whole fennel seeds chewed after the meal. If there is a lot of congestion, Ayurveda recommends favoring dry foods and astringent (puckering) tastes. Dry toast, apples, crackers, turmeric, and many raw vegetables are good for avoiding excess Kapha buildup and toning the digestive tract.

- Reduce sweetness. Kapha is the only dosha strongly identified with a taste—sweetness. Irrespective of calories, Kaphas will gain weight and go out of balance if there is too much sweet food in the diet. Avoiding ice cream, milk, sugary desserts, wheat bread, and butter (all considered sweet in Ayurveda) will often make a dramatic difference with the runny nose, blocked sinuses, allergies, and lethargy that Kaphas suffer from when out of balance. Over the long term, too much sweetness may help promote diabetes, a serious Kapha disease. Fortunately, there is one natural sweetener—raw honey—that is actually good for Kapha. Taking a tablespoon or two (but no more) every day helps release excess Kapha from the system.

- Stay warm. Being a cold dosha, Kapha benefits from heat. Dry heat is best if you are congested, a frequent Kapha complaint. Directing a sunlamp at your chest or using a heating pad under your back often helps with excess Kapha.

- Avoid dampness. Kapha is particularly sensitive to cold, damp conditions. Be careful not to expose your nose, throat, and lungs to cold winter air if you are feeling sick.

- Perform a dry massage on your body to stimulate circulation. This procedure is called *garshana* (page 133) and is done with special raw-silk gloves (available by mail order). You do not want to use oil when there is aggravated Kapha, since Kapha is an oily dosha. A brisk full-body rubdown, taking five to ten minutes, is good enough; do not work so hard that you tire yourself out. If you do not have gloves, a dry loofah sponge can substitute.

- Drink *warm* fluids during the day, but take them in moderation, since Kapha is already moist. To loosen congestion and ease sore throat, a tea made by boiling one-quarter teaspoon of dry ginger and turmeric in one cup of water is effective. A special Kapha-pacifying tea can also be mail-ordered. You can drink up to four cups a day.

- Exercise regularly, preferably every day. This is one of the best ways to avoid stagnation and the buildup of toxins in the body. Because they are generally strong and well muscled, Kaphas tend to be natural athletes when they are young; the arrival of adult responsibilities makes most Kaphas sedentary. That is a pity, for Kaphas benefit from exercise more than anyone else and should keep active at all ages.

- Be honest with yourself when you are sick and you need to recuperate. Kaphas have excellent stamina and enjoy physical activity; they also have a high threshold for pain and do not take to their beds unless they are very sick. If you are such a person, remember to take it easy when you feel sick enough to be in bed. You are probably twice as ill as most people. Kaphas can get quite gloomy unless they feel well cared for, so let your friends and family pay extra attention to you when you are low.

- Head congestion is a common Kapha problem, which can be forestalled by using a simple technique: Dissolve one-quarter teaspoon of salt in one-half cup of warm water. Standing over a sink, cup one hand with a little salt water in it. Close your left nostril, lean over, and inhale the water a few times through your right nostril so that it enters the sinuses. Close your right nostril and repeat on the other side. Do not inhale deeply (which will draw water into the lungs), or force your breath if your sinuses are clogged. You may sneeze or start to drain, which is good. Repeat two or three times as needed. This treatment is more effective after a warm shower has softened the sinus lining. If you feel any pain or have been diagnosed with a sinus infection, discontinue the treatment immediately. It is meant for keeping the nasal passages toned, not for curing a condition once it has developed.

HOW TO PERFORM GARSHANA

This dry massage should be done in the morning for 3 to 4 minutes before you take a bath and dress. Wearing the special silk gloves and using both hands, rub your skin quickly and fairly vigorously. Over the long bones of the arms and legs, use sweeping, back-and-forth strokes. Change to small, circular movements when you reach the joints—shoulders, elbows, wrists, etc. To begin with, 10 to 20 long strokes at a time are enough; this can be increased over time to as many as 40 strokes.

1. Start by massaging the head, using brisk circular motions, proceeding to long strokes as you reach the neck and shoulders. Now alternate these two movements as you continue down the arms: circular strokes

at the shoulder joint, long strokes down the upper arm, circular again at the elbows, long down the forearm, circular at the wrist, long down the hand, and finally circular strokes over the finger joints.

2. Moving to the chest, massage horizontally with long strokes, but avoid massaging directly over the heart and breasts.

3. Massage horizontally on the stomach for two strokes, then give two diagonal strokes. Using this alternating rhythm, proceed to the lower abdomen, lower back, buttocks, and thighs, giving added attention to any areas where there is extra fat. (This is to promote circulation in these areas and to loosen toxins associated with excess Kapha and fat.)

4. Stand up and massage the hip joints with circular motions. Now go down the legs as you did the arms: long strokes on the long leg bones, circular at the knees and ankles, ending with long strokes over the foot.

Garshana in combination with yoga exercises is particularly useful for getting rid of cellulite.

PART II

THE QUANTUM MECHANICAL HUMAN BODY

CHAPTER 6

QUANTUM MEDICINE FOR A QUANTUM BODY

On the never-ending journey of self-knowledge, the three doshas are an important landmark. They take us into the inner world, the only place where intelligence in all its forms—thoughts, emotions, drives, instincts, wishes, and beliefs—can be changed. But the doshas are only a halfway house. Beyond them lie even more profound revelations. In part II, I want to get to these greater depths by exploring the quantum mechanical human body—Ayurveda's term for the invisible software that shapes, controls, and creates the physical self.

In chapter 1 I stated some of the basic principles underlying the quantum mechanical body: it is a network of intelligence, the collected know-how not just of the brain but of the body's other 50 trillion cells; it responds immediately to our slightest thought and emotion, giving rise to the constant flow and change that is basic to our nature; it is not localized in space-time but is far more general, extending in all directions like a field. You cannot see your own quantum body, because it is made entirely of faint vibrations, fluctuations in the field, but you can be aware of it—indeed, your senses are keenly attuned to the quantum field, whose activity is more basic than either matter or energy. The fact that you can be aware of a level in nature 10 to 100 million times more subtle than the atom seems so surprising that I would like to expand on the notion.

EXPLORING THE INNER WORLD

You already know that the doshas are like a switching station where thoughts turn into matter. At first this seems impossible. Matter is solid and stable; it can be seen and touched, measured and weighed. Thoughts, on the other hand, are fleeting and invisible; they cannot be seen or touched, and measuring them (as with an electroencephalogram, or EEG), is an extremely crude affair. As one witty physiologist put it, understanding the brain with an EEG is like trying to understand the rules of football by sticking electrodes to the outside of the Astrodome and listening to the roar of the crowd.

Readings taken by looking into the skull are also distinctly limited. Thanks to the ultra-modern technology called PET (positron-emission tomography), it is now possible to image a single strong emotion or perception while a person is experiencing it. (This involves tracing patterns made by radioisotopes as the brain goes through the process of having a thought.) But these patterns, revealing as they are, do not tell us what kind of thought is being processed. You cannot tell love from hate; you cannot image the difference between a sane mind and an insane one, much less decode the incredible subtlety and miraculous variety of the mind body connection.

The only way truly to penetrate this realm is subjectively, from inside the quantum mechanical body. Here is where the trick of turning mind into matter is actually being managed. If meeting a snake in the woods frightens you, your heart starts to pound, your throat becomes dry, and your knees turn to rubber. By the time you jump back in fear, a split-second trans-formation has taken place inside you. Your mental impulse—totally abstract and nonmaterial—has manifested itself physically as molecules of adrenaline, which are concrete and totally material. The decision that makes this possible occurs subjectively; you choose to send a faint intention to your quantum mechanical body, and without hesitation it carries out its orders. Jumping back in fear is not your only option. If you were not afraid of snakes, there would be no adrenaline; instead, you might generate the chemicals that cause happiness and excitement, the thrill of discovery, or you might have a much more casual reaction altogether.

This opens the way for Ayurveda, which says that your mind gives you control, the ability to have *any* reaction you want. The great misfortune is that all of us are prepro-grammed along extremely rigid lines; we have only a few reactions instead of infinite ones. Because of that, we pay a price. The mind body connection ceases to be effortless and natural; stress starts to accumulate, and negative signals from the mind begin to damage the cells. An old Indian saying goes, "If you want to see what your thoughts were like yesterday, look at your body today. If you want to see what your body will be like tomorrow, look at your thoughts today." Most of us would be pretty upset to apply this test to ourselves. The real medicine our bodies need is medicine for our awareness.

QUANTUM MEDICINE

Once you know that there is a quantum body paralleling your physical one, many things make sense that were myster-ies before. Here are two tantalizing facts about heart attacks. Fact 1: More heart attacks occur at nine o'clock on Monday morning than at any other time of the week. Fact 2: The people who are least likely to suffer a fatal heart attack are those who report a high degree of job satisfaction.

Putting these two facts together, you begin to suspect that an element of choice is at work here. Although heart attacks are supposed to strike at random, it looks as if at least some heart attacks are controlled by the people having them. Certain people who hate their jobs get out of them on Monday morning by giving themselves a heart attack, while those who love their jobs do not. (Let's leave aside the question of why the job haters don't choose a less drastic outlet for their frustrations.) In conventional medicine, there is no known mechanism for giving yourself a heart attack using your mind. In Ayurveda's perspective, however, the heart is a printout of the same impulses that fill the mind, including the mind's disappointments, fears, and frustrations. At the quantum mechanical level, mind and body are united; therefore, it comes as no surprise that a deep, smoldering dissatisfaction lodged in the mind should express itself in a physical equivalent—a heart attack.

Indeed, any dissatisfaction *must* express itself physically, because all our thoughts turn into chemicals. When you are happy, chemicals in your brain travel throughout your body, telling every cell of your happiness. When they hear the message, the cells "get happy," too; that is, they begin to function more effectively by altering their own chemical processes. If you are depressed, on the other hand, the opposite happens. Your sadness is relayed chemically to each cell, causing a feeling of heartache, for example, and your immune system to grow weaker. Everything we think and do originates inside the quantum mechanical body and then bubbles up to the surface of life.

You have probably heard of experiments in which hypnotized subjects make their hands warmer, cause red patches to appear on their skin, or even raise blisters, just by the power of suggestion. This mechanism is not unique to hypnosis. We do the same thing all the time, only we do not usually have voluntary control over it. A typical heart-attack victim would be shocked to discover that he gave himself his attack. Yet, if you look beyond the grim implications, the really exciting news is that we have enormous, untapped powers. Instead of unconsciously creating disease, we could be consciously creating health.

❖

Because he is a doctor himself, Gerald Rice knows just how sick he is. After practicing internal medicine in Boston for twenty-five years, he was diagnosed at age 50 with chronic leukemia, or cancer of the blood's white cells. Gerald has been living in a mounting sense of panic for several months since he was diagnosed. Obsessed by his condition, he sits up at night poring over medical journals. What he reads is very discouraging. Patients with his form of leukemia usually live only a few years after the initial diagnosis.

It is still early. Gerald has noticed almost no symptoms other than feeling unusually tired during the day, but his white count is soaring above 40,000, more than four times the normal level, which is between 4,000 and 11,000. A leading cancer institute in New York City has urged him to try some new forms of chemotherapy, but he is apprehensive about exposing himself to the side effects of the medication when he currently has no symptoms. He has decided to wait despite the fact that going without treatment frightens him very much. A number of oncologists tell him the same thing: once his white counts get above 50,000, he must do something. Gerald lies awake at night fixated on this number; it is a frontier he dreads crossing.

Recently, having read of cancer cases that had progressed well under Ayurvedic treatment, he turned to us. Gerald's stance was very guarded, and his initial questions betrayed considerable anxiety about what he was getting himself into.

"What's your protocol for treating chronic leukemia?" he demanded immediately.

"This isn't a cancer clinic," he was told. "All our seriously ill patients begin with basically the same treatment."

This shocked him, since by his standards of practice, every specific variety of cancer merits its own intensive, narrowly focused approach. In Ayurveda we follow a different logic. Our goal is to reach the level of perfect balance that lies within every patient, no matter how sick. Experiencing this level brings healing, in and of itself, using the body's own methods.

"Right now your condition is dominated by feelings of dread and panic," he was told. "You are sending overwhelming signals of distress to your immune system, and you know as a physician that the immune response is extremely sensitive to such messages." He had to admit that this was true.

"What we want is to pull your awareness back to a healthier level, to a place where this disease is not so threatening. Ultimately, we would like you to find the place where it does not even exist."

Here he balked. "But it does exist; it *is* real. Are you asking me to be blind to that fact? If I am panicked, it's the leukemia that makes me feel that way," he protested. He began to become agitated. He had struggled to remain completely in control of himself ever since his devastating diagnosis. The prospect of changing his rigid, fearful stance was almost more frightening to him than his illness. We moved quickly to reassure him. Other kinds of medical treatments, either Ayurvedic or Western, would always be at his disposal. We would stay in consultation with his own physician and with top specialists in the Boston area. Without any treatment for his inner self, however, we did not consider that any outside medical treatment based on drugs or radiation went far enough.

In a serious or life-threatening illness, there can be many layers of imbalance concealing the depths where healing exists. Each layer is like a mask hiding the self from itself—one could spend a lifetime never suspecting that the quantum mechanical body exists. Perfect health is a reality at this deepest level, and it waits to be brought to the surface of life. The beginning of perfection, we tell our patients, is to let go of imperfection. For that, the Ayurvedic tradition has handed down many techniques, both physical and mental, for the physician to use.

"If you can pierce the mask of disease and contact your inner self, even for a few minutes a day, you will make tremendous strides toward healing," Gerald was told. "No one can guarantee your recovery, but this view of medicine is valid, and it works."

Gerald greeted these statements with a mixture of hopefulness and skepticism. I am keenly aware of the vulnerability that patients feel in this situation. They are prone to severe attacks of anxiety and guilt. They secretly wonder if they deserve their disease and therefore have unwittingly caused it; they blame themselves for not eating better, not visiting their doctor often enough, or not living more healthfully in general; they curse fate and yet beg it to reprieve them.

All of this anguish is unnecessary, and therefore, it does not have to be attacked head-on. The simple truth is that when a disease occurs, it brings a diseased reality with it, and the more serious the disease, the more distorted our view of reality is likely to become. For anyone in the grip of a truly debilitating illness, fear becomes dominant. That does not make it inevitable, however. Fear is the scenery you see when you are in a sick reality. If you change that reality, which is born inside yourself, the scenery will change, too.

"Tomorrow you can start the treatments," Gerald was told after his interview and initial physical. "You don't have to believe in them—all you have to do is experience them."

He sat quietly. "I'll try anything," he finally said in a low voice. He immediately checked into our Center. Considering all that he had been through, it was no surprise that Gerald's initial blood test, taken that afternoon, was dismal. His white count had soared to 52,000, well beyond what he had been led to think of as the point of no return.

Several things happened next. As soon as he arrived at the Center, Gerald was immersed in the routines for balancing the doshas that we covered in chapter 5. He was diagnosed as a Pitta type and placed on a Pitta-pacifying diet. Gerald's diet was strong on salads, fruits, rice, bread, and cold dishes, low on fats and salt, with an emphasis on sweet taste, all of which help relieve Pitta.

He learned meditation the first morning at the Center and began to meditate twice a day, just before breakfast and dinner. As a physician, Gerald was surprised by his surroundings. The Center is set in a very nourishing and life-supporting atmosphere. There is nothing conventionally medical about it. There is no somberness in the air, no antiseptic smells, no stark critical-care units with constantly beeping monitors.

Ayurveda encourages a natural setting, preferably a beautiful one, for recuperation. The five senses are constantly feeding signals to your quantum mechanical body, and each signal gets metabolized by you, entering your storehouse of sights, sounds, smells, and so on. If what the senses see, hear, touch, and smell reminds you of sickness, then something unhealthy is getting absorbed. How can you renew your reality if you are always subtly reminding yourself of the old one?

Gerald loved his long morning walks to the shore, but he was puzzled, too. "I don't see anything medical going on here," he protested from time to time. We asked him simply to continue his treatment.

The most active therapy Gerald underwent is called *panchakarma* (Sanskrit for "the five actions" or "the five treatments"), an extensive routine to purify the body of toxins that disease and improper diet have deposited. In Western medicine we know that waste products are continually building up in every cell of the body. These residues, resulting from oxidation caused by free radical molecules, are thought to play an active role in causing DNA to make mistakes (the cause of most cancers); almost certainly these wastes impair cell function, lead to more rapid aging, and ultimately kill our cells. What is not understood is exactly how this debris gets into the cells. Ayurveda says that it is the litter that imbalanced doshas leave behind, visible proof that some invisible process has gone wrong.

The Ayurvedic sages lumped all such toxic residues under the term *ama*, which they perceived as a foul-smelling, sticky, noxious substance that needs to be evacuated from the body as thoroughly as possible. Some purifying measures can be administered at home (as we will discuss later), but full-scale panchakarma is a specialized treatment, involving medical supervision as well as labor-intensive methods administered by Ayurvedic technicians.

Panchakarma doesn't push physical debris out of the cells, but it is said to push out the excess doshas, along with the ama that "sticks" to them, using the body's own channels of evacuation (sweat glands, urinary tract, intestines, and so on). From the patient's point of view, the daily massages and oil baths are extremely pleasant and very relaxing; from the quantum perspective, the channels that bring healing signals into our cells are being cleaned and restored. Panchakarma, I repeat, is not a cancer treatment. It is given to all patients in order to restore balance.

Within a day or two, Gerald felt the accumulated fatigue pouring out of his system, as if years of exhaustion were being drained away. Usually a driven and highly motivated person, he found he desperately needed long hours of rest and sleep. When he mentioned this, we told him that letting go of fatigue was the same as letting go of stress. Fatigue is the shadow of old stresses that build up in the nervous system. Being a doctor, Gerald was no stranger to stress, but his medical training denied that stress had anything to do with his illness.

I explained to him that his cells were imprinted with the memory of stress and over time lose their ability to function perfectly. Loops of intelligence get broken open, like disrupting an electrical circuit. The cell's overall intelligence weakens, and the final result is disease. In his case, the disease was leukemia; it could have been thousands of other disorders. The point is that the same intention applies to them all— restoring the body's own intelligence.

A week after he arrived, Gerald was ready to return home, still convinced that nothing medical had happened to him. In his final interview, he was presented with the results of a blood test taken that morning. According to the lab report, his white count had dropped by over 40 percent, from 52,000 to 28,000. He was astounded. This was a dramatic improvement. If Gerald had been taking conventional chemotherapy, a reduction of 10,000 in his counts over a few days would have been considered very encouraging.

Without any side effects, he felt healthier than he had in years, not just since he had been diagnosed with leukemia. Another serious symptom of his disease had disappeared entirely, the abnormal abundance of immature white cells produced by the bone marrow of leukemia patients. The blood smear taken on his first day had showed numerous abnormal cells; now there were none.

"This could be a fluke, couldn't it?" he asked. "The blood test can be wrong." But he knew that such routine tests are highly likely to be right—he relies on them every day in his own practice.

THE POWER OF AWARENESS

I believe the secret to Gerald's recovery was a change in his awareness. He learned that there is more self-control in letting go than in trying to control one's body by force. The follow-up period proved this point dramatically. After he left the Center, Gerald threw himself back into his work, subjecting himself to the usual heavy stress, and on his next visit three months later, his white-cell count had zoomed back up to over 45,000. He plunged into depression, but with the Ayurvedic treatments his counts came back down again. Immensely relieved and grateful, he went home and pitched himself into his old life even more furiously. Not surprisingly, the counts rose a third time.

When he returned for another week of treatment, I said something he didn't expect: "There's a lot of pain whenever you go home, isn't there?"

"What do you mean?" he asked guardedly. "It's true that I'm sick."

"I mean beyond your being sick."

He didn't say anything. It seemed highly significant that his leukemia had been diagnosed just four months after his wife had died of a heart attack in her mid-fifties. Gerald missed his wife terribly. Moreover, when he came home at night, there was friction with his divorced daughter, who had moved in to take care of him.

What he had to recognize was that his condition was related to his state of awareness. His mind was deeply influencing his body. "Imagine that your awareness is like a violin string. The string can play any kind of note, high or low, depending on where you place your finger. Right now, you are putting out all kinds of missed notes. Not just your runaway white counts, but your mood swings, your nervous expectations, your pain and grief, are all notes coming out of the same position.

"In conventional medicine, only the notes count. A huge amount of energy is spent killing the abnormal white cells. But it is equally important that you change your position on the string. Then you would be creating a new reality, complete with new notes. Isn't that what we have been doing all along? Think about it."

Gerald admitted that he felt better every day he spent at the Center and worse every day he spent at home. "But you're not saying that feeling good makes leukemia regress, are you?" he demanded.

"If feeling good is part of healing, then yes, that is what I am saying. It's not really a matter of your moods. Naturally your moods swing during the course of a serious illness—you can feel happy or despondent, hopeful or hopeless without warning.

"Underlying these unpredictable mood swings is your quantum level of awareness, which has become disturbed. Changes in this level of awareness are what bring about changes in mood; if your deep awareness shifts, your moods will follow like a weather vane. We should also expect to see similar indications in your body, and your altered blood counts are a good example. Change in awareness is terribly important. As a doctor, you can't have it only one way and say that negative emotions disturb the immune system. It must also be true that positive states of awareness will help you to get well."

Gerald thought that this was reasonable. Weighed against his conventional medical training, which led him to be skeptical about any sort of "mind over matter" in the healing process, he had to set his own vivid, undeniable experience. Our conversation took place several months ago. He continues to benefit from the approach outlined here, but it is taking time for Gerald to break out of his old patterns completely. We think he has turned the corner, though. There is much less evidence of a struggle on his part. One of his most cherished beliefs, that he must fight for life with every atom of his being, is giving way. Now he is starting to accept the possibility of a very profound Ayurvedic truth: if you can let go of imperfection, perfection will appear by itself.

CHAPTER 7

OPENING THE CHANNELS OF HEALING

Getting back in touch with the quantum mechanical body is the most important goal in Ayurveda. We call this process "quantum healing." As understood by modern medicine, the body's healing abilities are nearly infinite, but quantum healing *is* infinite. The flow of intelligence bubbling up from the quantum mechanical body can be channeled in countless ways to achieve any result in the physical body, including the cure of serious, life-threatening diseases and the reversal of the aging process itself.

All of these things will be laid out in detail in the following pages, as we discuss the major healing techniques of Ayurveda. All are medical techniques used in our Center, but most also have home versions that you can learn from this book or from a few hours of instruction from a qualified *Creating Health* educator. The term "healing technique" should be understood in its broadest sense, applying to anyone who wants to come closer to perfect health, not just the sick. The seven techniques to be covered are:

Panchakarma   *Marma Therapy*
Meditation   *Aromatherapy*
Healing Sounds   *Music Therapy*
Healing Visualization

PANCHAKARMA—PURIFICATION OF THE BODY

Physical impurities play a large part in hiding our perfect nature from ourselves, like dust on a mirror. But such impurities lie much deeper than dust, and they have more than physical effects: one's entire psychology is linked to one's physical condition. The value of panchakarma is that it offers a systematic treatment for dislodging and flushing toxins from every cell, using the same organs of elimination that the body naturally employs—sweat glands, blood vessels, urinary tract, and intestines.

The ancient texts praise panchakarma as a seasonal treatment for ensuring balance year in and year out. Despite a high standard of health that keeps most of us feeling healthy most of the time, Americans generally do not reach old age free of disease. Indeed, less than a third of old people show no sign of cancer, heart disease, arthritis, diabetes, osteoporosis, and other degenerative disorders endemic to old age. All these diseases lack a specific cause; in the eyes of a Western doctor, they are complex disorders that accumulate over a lifetime, rather like a rolling snowball accumulating tiny flakes of snow. No single snowflake is the cause of the snowball, yet with each flake, the snowball gets bigger and bigger. In terms of the body, the snowflakes are tiny bits of ama, and we cannot think of being in perfect balance unless these are removed as fast as they are picked up.

STEPS OF PANCHAKARMA

Although literally translated as "the five actions," pan-chakarma actually involves a series of steps tailored to body type and requiring supervision over the course of about a week. It has taken approximately five years to clarify these procedures and adapt them for use in the West. As with other aspects of traditional Ayurveda, panchakarma has been hampered by confusion and by different modes of practice throughout India. At the Chopra Center, panchakarma follows these steps:

Oleation (snehana). The patient takes sesame seeds or herbalized ghee (clarified butter) for several mornings in a row to soften up the doshas and minimize digestive action. (In Ayurvedic terms, one is temporarily quieting down the *agni*, or digestive fire.)

Laxative (virechana). A gentle laxative, such as senna, is taken to flush out the intestinal tract, lowering Pitta and further bringing down agni.

Oil massage (abhyanga). Technicians administer a full-body abhyanga like the one done at home in the daily routine but about twice as long and much more thorough. The oil is herbalized according to body type. More force is used to loosen the excess doshas and direct them toward the organs of elimination. There is also a related treatment called *shirodhara*, in which warm, herbalized sesame oil is dripped in a stream onto the forehead to profoundly relax the nervous system and balance Prana Vata, the subdosha of Vata that exerts major control over the brain.

Sweat treatments (swedana). Herbalized steam opens up the pores and begins to rid the body of impurities through the sweat glands.

Enema (basti). Medicated enemas, of which Ayurveda lists well over a hundred, are used for various specific reasons; in general, this treatment is used to flush the loosened doshas out through the intestinal tract.

Nasal administrations (nasya). Medicinal oils or herbal mixtures are inhaled, clearing the sinus passages, draining excess mucus, and decreasing accumulated Kapha, which tends to build up in the head.

The following two case studies may give you a better idea of how effective these procedures can be:

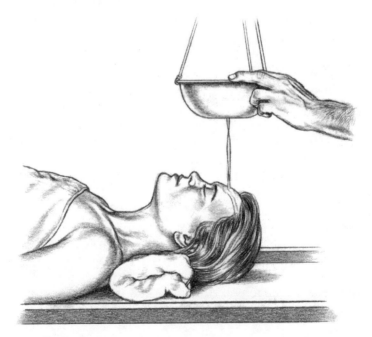

Shirodhara profoundly soothes the nervous system.

❖

Daniel Frazier, a contractor in his late forties, began suffering recurrent lower back pains ten years ago. As frequently happens, his doctors found it difficult to isolate a cause for his pain; although agonizingly real to him, the scans of his back revealed nothing problematic. After consulting a number of specialists, he resigned himself to living with chronic pain. When an attack occurred, he stayed home in bed and lived on muscle relaxants until it passed.

An Ayurvedically trained doctor examined Daniel and informed him that his pain appeared to be due to an imbalance of Apana Vata, the subdosha of Vata that controls the lower back and intestinal tract. A Vata-pacifying routine was prescribed, along with a week of panchakarma and yoga classes. By the end of the treatment, his pain had disappeared completely for the first time in a decade. Since then, Daniel has suffered little or no pain at all; he returns periodically for additional panchakarma to prevent any possible recurrence of his condition.

❖

Cheryl De Luca fell into a typical adolescent pattern when she began to develop acne at age 17; when it was still present at age 31, however, it was definitely not typical. Fortunately her skin outbreaks were relatively mild and not permanently disfiguring. Still, living with chronic acne was difficult for her and had made her feel very self-conscious. As often happens, over-the-counter remedies had been of little use; curtailing chocolate, tomatoes, fried foods, and other suspicious foods made little impact.

When she was in her mid-twenties, Cheryl's dermatologist put her on tetracycline, an antibiotic widely prescribed for adult acne. She experienced occasional, mild side effects, namely upset stomachs and sensitivity to bright sunlight. These were a small price to pay, her doctor reasoned, for controlling the disease. On the other hand, Cheryl was bothered by the idea of taking daily antibiotics indefinitely. When she consulted our Center her condition was diagnosed as Pitta imbalance. (One of Pitta's five subdoshas, Bhrajaka Pitta, gives luster to the skin when in balance, but is often responsible for skin problems if out of balance.)

Treatment was very simple. Cheryl was put on a Pitta-pacifying diet and instructed in the Ayurvedic daily routine. She went through panchakarma for a week at the Center. Her acne began to subside and disappeared entirely within six months. She has now been free of her condition and off medication for a year.

PANCHAKARMA TODAY

In India today, seasonal panchakarma treatment is the province of the rich and of those few who have adhered faithfully to Ayurvedic tradition. The classic texts, however, clearly state that everyone needs panchakarma. Three times a year is best, ideally at the turn of spring, fall, and winter. Taking panchakarma as an inpatient is also recommended, since the body gets deeper rest if you do not have to travel to and from a clinic every day. However, outpatient treatment is extremely effective. As a minimum, you should try to take one week of panchakarma every year if you are in good health. Sick patients should take outpatient panchakarma only under the advice of a physician trained in Ayurveda. Also, unless a physician recommends it, panchakarma is not routinely given to children under the age of 12.

MEDITATION—A TECHNIQUE FOR "GOING BEYOND"

Physical impurities in cells have their equivalents in the mind: fear, anger, greed, compulsiveness, doubt, and other negative emotions. Operating at the quantum level, they can be as damaging to us as any chemical toxin. As we saw, the mind body connection turns negative attitudes into chemical toxins, the so-called "stress hormones" that have been linked to many different diseases. Ayurveda lumps all negative tendencies together as "mental ama," which needs to be cleaned from the mind. But how?

It is not possible to purify the mind by thinking about it. An angry mind cannot conquer its own anger; fear cannot quench fear. Instead, a technique is required that goes beyond the domain where fear, anger, and all other forms of mental ama hold sway. This technique is meditation. If properly taught and used, meditation allows a person to become unstuck from the ama in his thoughts and emotions. In our Center, we prescribe Primordial Sound Meditation, or PSM, as a simple, natural way of accomplishing this goal.

As a young physician in the 1970s, I was attracted to meditation for two reasons, one personal, the other professional. The personal reason was the promise of inner growth, of reaching an expanded state of mental and spiritual development. The professional reason was the large body of research on meditation that established that this meditation was "real," that is, it produced tangible benefits.

Meditation is not forcing your mind to be quiet; it's finding the quiet that is already there. In fact, when you examine the background static of worry, resentment, wishful thinking, fantasy, unfulfilled hopes, and vague dreams in your head, it becomes clear that the internal dialogue going on inside is literally controlling us. Each of us is the victim of memory—

that's how the Ayurvedic masters diagnosed it thousands of years ago.

Behind the screen of our internal dialogue, there is something entirely different: the silence of a mind that is not imprisoned by the past. That is the silence we want to bring into our awareness through meditation. Why is this important? Because silence is the birthplace of happiness. Silence is where we get our bursts of inspiration, our tender feelings of compassion and empathy, our sense of love. These are all delicate emotions and the chaotic roar of the internal dialogue easily drowns them out. But when you discover the silence in your mind, you no longer have to pay attention to all those random images that trigger worry, anger, and pain.

If you are going to pursue the full spiritual benefits of meditation, I recommend you seek out a qualified teacher whose spiritual tradition you respect. But at the same time, there are meditative techniques for reaching your inner silence that you can learn right now, because they're basically physiological. They take advantage of the natural silence that exists in the mind body system when it's relaxed.

When you're ready to begin, sit quietly holding your hands lightly at your side or in your lap. Now, with your eyes closed, start to breathe lightly and easily. Let your attention easily follow your breathing. Feel your breath entering your nostrils and flowing down into your lungs. Don't inhale deeply or hold your breath, just breathe normally. When you exhale, let your attention follow the air up out of the lungs and softly through the nostrils.

Nothing is forced here. The breath is moving easily and gently, your attention is following it softly as leaves swaying in the treetops. As your breathing relaxes, make it a little lighter. Again, don't force this, but when you feel that your

breathing wants to get a bit shallower and lighter, just le. ..
happen. If you start to feel short of breath, don't worry. This
means that you need a little more air and that deep stresses are
coming out. Or you might also be forcing your breathing to be
lighter than it wants to be. Return to whatever rate of breathing your body feels comfortable with.

When you are comfortable with this effortless process, you
can add the mantra "so hum" to the procedure, silently thinking the word "so" on each inhalation and "hum" on each
exhalation.

Continue this exercise for two to five minutes, just closing
your eyes and focusing your mind on easy, natural breathing
and silently repeating "so hum" with each cycle of your
breath.

What is happening with this exercise? You probably noticed
that just by paying attention to your breathing you sank
deeper and deeper into relaxation, and as you did so, your
mind naturally became quieter. Did you sense that? If so, you
probably experienced a few glimpses of complete silence,
which you aren't likely to have noticed, because I didn't ask
you to be on the lookout. If you had looked for silence it
wouldn't have appeared. Yet I imagine there were stretches
where you lost track of time, which is a good indication that
you were getting very near to the goal. Most people experience much fainter thoughts than usual, which is another
good sign.

As you gain experience with meditation, you'll begin to feel
the reappearance of youthful energy and vitality that is being
released from a deeper level of the nervous system. This is a
very profound change and the real fountain of youth.

Although meditation has been wrapped in an aura of mysti-
cism for many centuries, at its heart lies this extremely practical

and unmystical process of quieting the mind. It is the surest way to open a channel of healing.

THE MIND HEALS ITSELF

Matt's life changed profoundly in his last year of high school, when his parents began to go through an acrimonious divorce. All through school he had been a high achiever, capable of getting A's with minimal effort; on the strength of his academic record, he had won a full scholarship to MIT. His parents had always doted on Matt. Their decision to divorce was difficult for everyone in the family; Matt remembers lying in bed hearing his parents' violent arguments through the wall.

As these arguments continued, he began to develop headaches. Instead of feeling bright and focused all the time, Matt noticed that he fell into stretches of depression. He left for college, but separation from home made his symptoms worse. His headaches became blindingly severe, causing acute pain, dizziness, and vomiting. His depression deepened, and before the first semester was over, he had to drop out. He could hardly concentrate well enough to read a newspaper or listen to music.

Matt moved in with his father, a prominent lawyer who was bitterly disappointed over what had happened to his son. He hired Matt to work as a clerk in his firm and sent him to psychiatrists, who tried couch therapy as well as antidepressants. Nothing worked very well or for very long. Medical treatment for the headaches was also unsuccessful. By the time he was 21 Matt was still so depressed that he had to struggle against thoughts of suicide.

At this point he heard about meditation through a friend; his doctor agreed that it might be helpful and advised him to try it. Matt learned that meditation is a purely mechanical technique employed for twenty minutes morning and evening. He was given a *mantra*, selected not for its meaning but strictly for its sound. That sound alone attracts the mind and leads it, effortlessly and naturally, to ever more subtle levels of the thinking process.

As the mantra comes and goes in one's awareness, it begins to seek still subtler levels of thought until eventually all thought is left behind. At this point we say that the mind has transcended. Because it is no longer caught up in thoughts of any kind, the mind is exposed to its own deepest nature, to pure awareness. The silence of pure awareness is extremely refreshing to the mind, which finds it increasingly easy not to cling to old thought patterns; rigid habits of thinking and feeling begin to fall away of their own accord. When this happens, the mind is actually learning to heal itself.

The first few times Matt meditated, he in fact began to notice a distinct change in his mental state. Small islands of clarity began to appear, in which he felt completely alert, free of dullness or depression, and infused with happiness. Over time the islands grew bigger and bigger; Matt lived for the moments when he found them. However, the islands of clarity were restricted to his meditations. When he was active, his depression returned at full force. After a few months he consulted me.

"What you are experiencing," I said, "are different levels of awareness. Your depression is on one level, your headaches on another, your islands of clarity on another still. Meditation is taking you deeper and deeper inside yourself, until you reach the area untouched by illness. This is a very real part of yourself.

"As you keep meditating, these moments of clarity will expand and become the norm. Right now, you are fixated on certain patterns in your awareness, and your body knows it. Your depression has captured your attention, which is why you find it difficult if not impossible to focus on other things.

"But as you have seen, you can let go. Meditation is a kind of letting go, allowing yourself simply to be. And when you permit that to happen, your attention will always fly back to the silent, peaceful, unchanging level we simply call the self. The self is home base for the mind, and by returning to it, you infuse your mind with the same peace and silence."

I drew a simple diagram.

"Using the technique of meditation, one takes the mind out of activity into silence. After a few seconds or minutes, the mind will naturally come back up, like a diver bobbing back

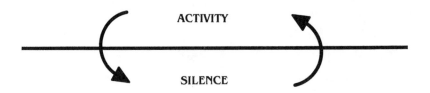

up to the surface of the water. What brings it back? The same impulses that guide us every day—our desires. A faint desire causes a ripple of activity inside the silence, this ripple expands, and eventually you have a full-blown thought.

"However, this thought is not the same as before. It will have an aura of happiness and freshness, just because you have fetched it from a deeper level of yourself."

Matt mentioned that recently a new phenomenon had begun. When he felt a moment of clarity, he would suddenly envision lines of verse. These formed a complete poem, which was not coming to him word by word or even by the ordinary process of thinking. It simply appeared.

"That's a good sign," I said. "As you get closer to your own creative center, your whole style of thinking is changing. In place of bits and pieces, things appear as a whole. In place of troubling conflicts, there is no conflict. The self is a different landscape, new scenery for the mind to absorb. As long as you are in that landscape, you will experience yourself as completely different."

In a gentle tone I added, "The intense suffering you experience in your mind is a distraction from reality. The reality is that you can go to these peaceful islands anytime you want. They are permanent parts of yourself; if you lived on them permanently, there would be no way for depression to touch you. What meditation is teaching you is that reality, in the sense of wholeness, has a powerful pull. It is trying to call you home. You are already beginning to trust this process, aren't you?"

Matt admitted that he was, adding that his headaches had decreased considerably, and that he had begun to see the possibility of actually turning his attention to his lifelong dream of becoming a writer.

"That trust is another good sign," I said. "You are remembering yourself. Finding your true self is a very profound process, which has no end. Your body is listening to healthier signals now, and as long as you continue to take your mind back to its source, over and over, the signals will get even healthier. You've made a breakthrough; getting well is just a matter of time."

MEDITATION AS MEDICINE

This is an encouraging story from one patient, but the application of meditation to large-scale disorders is also highly promising. One of the best examples is high blood pressure, or hypertension, the infamous "silent killer" that has almost no symptoms and yet is implicated in the vast majority of heart attacks and strokes.

As many as a third of American adults fall into the borderline hypertensive range; an estimated 30 million have already been warned by their doctors and yet take no treatment. Borderline hypertension often responds extremely well to meditation. This was first established by a 1974 study conducted at Harvard Medical School. Twenty-two hypertensive patients were measured twelve hundred times, both before and after they learned to meditate. Over a period ranging from one month to five years, their average readings dropped from 150/94 to 141/88. This was enough to bring the lower number (diastolic pressure) back from borderline to an acceptable reading; it did not lower the upper number (systolic pressure) quite enough—120 or 130 is considered normal here—but at least there was significant improvement. These results, subsequently repeated in many other studies, were independent of whether the subjects took blood-pressure medication.

You may think that reducing mild hypertension is not a great achievement, yet even a small rise in blood pressure is considered extremely dangerous in the long run. Half of all deaths associated with hypertension fall into the borderline range. Insurance companies use blood pressure as the most significant indicator of life expectancy. A middle-aged man with normal blood pressure (120/80) is expected to live sixteen years longer than someone with moderate hypertension (150/100). Just by practicing meditation, most people under the age of 40 could expect to fall below the limit set for borderline hypertension, which is 130/90.

Meditating can also lower abnormally high cholesterol levels. Cholesterol is a primary risk factor for heart attacks, because excess cholesterol in the blood is directly linked to the fatty plaque deposits that clog the arteries leading to the heart.

On the surface, it seems amazing that the mind could control serum cholesterol. Your serum cholesterol is determined by a complex interplay of diverse factors, all of them physical: diet, age, heredity, digestive efficiency, and liver function all play an important part. Several years ago two researchers in Israel, M. J. Cooper and M. M. Aygen, selected twenty-three patients with elevated cholesterol levels; twelve were taught meditation and practiced it for eleven months, while the remaining eleven did not.

At the end of that time, the meditating group showed a marked drop in their cholesterol levels, from an average of 255 to 225 (a reading of 200 is considered ideal for adults in the United States). The nonmeditators did not show a significant decrease. The subjects were screened so that age, diet, weight, and exercise were not factors. Similar reductions were obtained in a separate study by the same team, this time showing that cholesterol could be lowered in people who had more normal cholesterol readings.

These findings suggest that the entire mind body system can be influenced by a single mental technique, and indeed the encouraging results with hypertension and cholesterol were recently expanded to cover many other diseases. Dr. David Orme-Johnson, a research psychologist, examined the health of two thousand meditators. All the subjects Orme-Johnson selected belonged to a group health insurance policy for meditators. To qualify, each person signed a piece of paper stating that he practiced meditation regularly; they also agreed to be checked periodically to ensure that they were meditating correctly. A major national carrier who covered hundreds of other groups underwrote this policy. There were no prerequisites about diet or lifestyle.

Orme-Johnson wanted to see how often a typical meditator went to the doctor compared to the average person. The difference turned out to be quite startling. Meditators went for outpatient treatment:

46.8 percent less often if they were children (0–19 years)

54.7 percent less often if they were young adults (19–39 years)

73.7 percent less often if they were older adults (40 and over)

This represents a striking improvement in health. A middle-aged meditator, for example, would visit his doctor once for every four times an average person went. The fact that older people benefited most is also highly significant. Turning to specific illnesses, the study found that heart attacks and cancer, the two leading causes of death in America, were reduced far below the norm. Meditators had:

87.3 percent fewer admissions to the hospital for heart disease

55.4 percent fewer admissions for benign and malignant tumors of all types

No one has seen reductions like this with the use of conventional prevention techniques. If a cholesterol-reducing drug could decrease heart attacks by 50 percent it would make worldwide headlines (obviously, this has not happened). This is doubly true for the cancer figures. Any reduction in this field would be a major breakthrough. After fifty years of massively funded research, the average cancer rates in the United States remain essentially unchanged, and the length of time that patients survive their diagnoses of cancer has barely budged for most types of malignancies. (This speaks for all patients as a whole; individuals of course may do better than indicated by the statistics and with certain types of cancers, such as childhood leukemia and localized breast cancer, medicine has made great progress.)

To get a fair comparison, Orme-Johnson used 600,000 members of the same health insurance carrier. He examined all the claims filed over a five-year period to ensure that he was not seeing a short-term deviation from normal. In all, the average meditator, whether child, young adult, or elderly, saw a doctor half as often as the average American.

How to Learn to Meditate

Because it is a subtle and specialized technique, meditation is best learned from a qualified instructor; it is not as easy to learn it properly from a book. Through the Chopra Center, we have certified over five hundred teachers of Primordial Sound Meditation. The cost of instruction is $225 for adults, in line with other self-development programs. Qualified instruction ensures that the technique is taught correctly in every detail and is tailored to your individual needs.

I recommend that you start with the simple breathing awareness meditation technique described on page 158. Once you taste the benefits of quieting the mind, seek out a qualified meditation teacher so you are certain you are practicing meditation correctly. Information on how to locate a certified Primordial Sound Meditation teacher is provided in Appendix A.

HEALING SOUNDS—NATURE'S FINEST VIBRATIONS

Nature provides a wide variety of vibrations to remind us of our essential nature. Any sound that helps to quiet and expand the mind can be considered a healing sound. According to Ayurveda, these subtle sounds are not incidental: all of nature is made up of them. In the complete stillness of the quantum mechanical universe, primordial sounds are born, form patterns, and in time blossom into matter, energy, and all the infinite variety of things made of matter and energy— stars, trees, rocks, and human beings. The calls of wild birds, the buzzing of bees, the crash of waves against the shore, the rustling of leaves in a summer breeze—all of these sounds can be healing. Make it a point to spend time in nature and listen to the healing sounds that surround you. If you live in a dense urban environment where you cannot regularly access natural sounds, bring nature to you with recordings of rain forests, ocean waves, or waterfalls. The theory behind healing sound treatment is that the mind can return to the quantum level, introduce certain sounds that may have become distorted somewhere along the line, and thus have a profound healing influence in the body. Connecting to these healing sounds on a regular basis is good medicine.

QUANTUM REALITY

Since this is such a foreign concept to people rooted in material reality, as all of us are, let's take a moment to put primordial sound into perspective. Western physicists already acknowledge that at the deepest level of the natural world we find the quantum field. A quantum is defined as the smallest unit of light, electricity, or other energy that can possibly exist. (The word *quantum* comes from the Latin for "how much?") Quantum reality defies our commonsense notions. There is no solid matter in it, for example. An atom used to be considered the smallest particle of matter in creation. The word *atom* in fact comes from the Greek for "not able to be divided." Yet, up close an atom is composed of tinier bits of matter whirling at lightning speed around a huge empty space—so empty that it rivals the void of intergalactic space; the interval between two electrons is proportionately wider than the one separating the earth and the sun.

If you zero in on these bits of subatomic matter, they are not material at all but rather mere vibrations of energy that have taken on the appearance of solidity. This discovery, that matter is a fluctuation of energy dressed up in a different guise, fueled the quantum revolution led by Einstein and his colleagues at the beginning of the last century. Instead of relying on solid particles that move around like billiard balls on a table, physicists were confronted with ghostly vibrations that looked substantial one minute and abstract the next.

The quantum revolution made it inevitable that our worldview would change. Quantum physics proved that the infinite variety of objects we see around us—stars, galaxies, mountains, trees, butterflies, and amoebas—is connected by infinite, eternal, unbounded quantum fields, a kind of invisible quilt that has all of creation stitched into it. Objects that look separate and distinct to us are in fact all sewn into the design of this vast quilt. The hard edges of any object, such as a chair or table, are an illusion forced upon us by the limits of our sight. If we had eyes tuned to the quantum world, we would see these edges blur and finally melt, giving way to unlimited quantum fields. Finding this quantum level of nature has had practical applications; it gave us X rays, transistors, superconductors, and lasers, things that were inconceivable until science delved deeper into the fabric of creation.

It is now believed that a single superfield, called the unified field, exists; it is the ultimate reality that underlies all of nature. Like a tree whose twigs lead to stems, stems to branches, and branches to one main trunk, the whole multiplicity of nature comes together in this one all-embracing field. Since we too are part of nature, we must be part of the unified field. It is in and around us all the time.

It is possible to experience this all-encompassing field in your own mind, via meditation. A meditator describes the experience:

> I feel the boundaries of the mind being pushed out, like the ever-widening circumference of a circle, until the circle disappears and only infinity remains. It is a feeling of great freedom, but also one of naturalness, far more real and natural than being confined to a small space.

This is surely a dramatic shift of awareness, which causes the mind to grasp a new, profound truth—that a human being is more than a package of flesh and blood localized in time and space. In fact we have two homes, one local, the other infinite. If you turn to physics, you find that in the world of our senses, electrons, quarks, and other elementary particles also appear to be localized in time and space. But once you venture over the quantum threshold, each particle is the tip of a wave that extends infinitely in all directions through space-time. This means that you cannot see yourself accurately until you become aware of both your identities.

The same meditator continues:

> Sometimes the sense of infinity is so strong that I lose the sensation of body or matter in an infinite, unbounded awareness, an eternal, never-changing continuum of consciousness.

It is highly unlikely that this description is just a subjective illusion. Countless others like it have been recorded in every spiritual tradition of man, both Eastern and Western.

SOUND AS MEDICINE

The obvious question arises: How are we connected to the unified field? By invisible "threads" composed of faint vibrations, what Ayurveda calls primordial sound. This again is plausible from the viewpoint of a modern physicist. It is obvious that when two electrons are held together in a helium atom despite the immense void that separates them, an invisible but extremely strong bond is present. This bond must also have an element of design in it, since every atom in the universe is perfect and remains perfect forever.

The sages of Ayurveda claimed to have detected these bonds, which act as the glue of the universe, through sounds that came into their own awareness. Having heard them, the sages could also reproduce these sounds and pass them on to others. A primordial sound can be spoken or chanted aloud; it is more powerful still if used internally, as a mental sound. The proof that primordial sound is real lies in its application. If the body is basically glued together by sounds, as the sages contend, then the presence of a disease means that some sounds must have gone out of tune.

❖

Not until she turned 75 did Molly Sanders have any trouble with her heart. She began to suffer from recurrent bouts of dull chest pain that were diagnosed as angina pectoris. Molly did not have to exert herself to bring on an attack—one might come when she was sitting still, or it might wake her up in the middle of the night.

Her diary records fifteen episodes between January and May when the angina began, or about three attacks per month. Some were mild and passed after one or two minutes, others were more severe, emanating pain from the center of her chest for up to ten minutes, leaving her panting and feeling faint. "I didn't live this long by worrying about my problems," she told her friends. Nonetheless, the experience frightened her.

When she went to her cardiologist, Molly's tests disclosed no serious blockage in her coronary arteries. Like most elderly people, her arteries had hardened somewhat, but there were no large fatty plaque deposits starving the heart muscle of oxygen. However, there is a second kind of angina that results from spasms of the coronary vessels, and Molly had that. Her arteries were just narrow enough that mild, even unnoticeable stress tightened them sufficiently to bring on an angina attack.

"We don't know everything about this condition," her doctor said. "Just take it easy from now on."

"When you're seventy-five years old," Molly snapped, "all you do is take it easy."

Although she began taking a standard medication to stabilize her blood vessels, she wanted to do everything possible to avoid taking medicines on a long-term basis. Early in June, on the advice of her son, Molly became our patient. After taking a complete medical history, we instructed her in meditation and encouraged her to begin listening to the sounds of nature on a daily basis.

We then taught her to chant aloud the sound associated with the heart center. According to Tantra, a spiritual tradition that is closely related to Ayurveda, we each possess seven energy centers known as *chakras*. These chakras can be thought of as junction points between mind and matter.

The first center at the base of the spine is associated with basic survival issues. The second center in the reproductive area governs creativity. The third located in the solar plexus is concerned with personal power. The fourth center in the heart is important in relationships. The fifth chakra, located in the throat, is responsible for expressing ourselves. The sixth chakra is located between the eyes (usually known as the "third eye") and is the center for insight and intuition. Finally, the seventh center is at the crown of the head and is said to open when we experience higher states of consciousness.

Each chakra has a mantra associated with it. According to Tantra expressing the mantra with your attention in the chakra can open up energy that may be congested in that region.

The mantras for each of the seven energy centers are as follows:

Chakra	*Location*	*Mantra*
1st Chakra	Base of Spine	Lam
2nd Chakra	Genital	Vam
3rd Chakra	Solar plexus	Ram
4th Chakra	Heart	Yum
5th Chakra	Throat	Hum
6th Chakra	Third eye	Sham
7th Chakra	Crown	Om

We encouraged Molly to chant the sound for the heart chakra several times per day. Two months later, Molly wrote me a happy letter that began, "I have no more pain!" Her angina attacks had stopped a week after she began using the heart chakra mantra and have not returned. Delight and relief came through in her writing. She feels comfortable in activity now—most angina sufferers are extremely anxious about exerting themselves, even slightly. This summer she took a bold step and enrolled as a full-time college student. She tells me with pride that she is the oldest undergraduate in the history of her college.

How does Ayurveda explain the effects of using sounds to heal? Intellectually, you cannot possibly analyze all the vibrations that influence your life. The oscillation of the atoms comprising your cells, the beating of your heart, the rhythms of the planets—each of these influence your life in subtle but profound ways. According to Ayurveda the many different vibrations that comprise our lives sometimes get "out of synch." This disharmony that results sows the seeds for illness.

In that event, Ayurveda tells us to apply a specifically chosen sound, like a mold or template slipped over the disturbed cells coaxing them back into line, not physically, but by repairing the sequence of sound at the heart of every cell. In the case of a disorder like angina, we know that the brain sends specific signals that constrict the arteries, working through messenger molecules that stimulate nerve and muscle cells in the middle layers of the blood vessels. Molly's spasms were being caused by some kind of improper message. Certain medicines take advantage of this fact by inhibiting the brain's chemical messengers so that their message never gets delivered. But the real source of these molecules is the mind; if one went directly to the thinking process and corrected the brain's impulses, then treatment should be even more effective and gentler. This is the purpose of healing sounds.

The degree of healing achieved by sound varies from person to person. After several years of prescribing them, we have witnessed hundreds of cases where patients with heart disease, cancer, multiple sclerosis, and even AIDS have reported alleviation of pain, anxiety, and various other troubling symptoms. These are all anecdotal reports, meaning that they have not been studied statistically using the proper controls needed for scientific validation. Therefore, they cannot be offered as proof that this subtle healing technique is effective; by the standards of scientific medicine, there is a long way to go before ironclad proof is available. On the other hand, the Ayurvedic approach is rooted in thousands of years of experience, and using it can supplement the benefits of standard medical treatment.

Discovering that the human body is fundamentally a web of sound comes as a revelation, and when put into practice, the theory yields remarkable results. In a matter of a few hours, one's self-image completely changes; people often report dramatic transformations in their powers of perception. Using a healing sound is a perfect illustration of the Ayurvedic saying that "the world is as you are." When your perception opens up "in here," so does everything "out there."

HEALING VISUALIZATION—USING ATTENTION AND INTENTION

Focusing your attention on an area in your body that needs healing and introducing an intention is a powerful therapeutic technique. Ayurveda says, "Whatever we put our attention on grows stronger in our lives." If you spend two hours a day at the fitness center building up your body, your muscles will grow but your grades in school may fall. If you spend your evenings and weekends at the office, your business may grow but your family relationships may suffer.

Ayurveda states that you can use your attention to activate healing in your body. You can change your mind and body by consciously directing your awareness to the aspect you believe needs attention.

Another principle of Ayurveda is, "Intention has infinite organizing power." This means that just being clear on a desired outcome can have a pronounced effect on achieving your goal, without necessarily having to handle all the details. When you want to throw a baseball, you do not have to analyze the contraction and release of every muscle in your body—you simply have the intention and your inner intelligence coordinates the tens of millions of activities that need to occur for you to throw the ball. The release of sugar from your liver, the metabolism of the sugar into energy, changes in blood flow, and your breathing pattern are organized by nature without your conscious control. If you had to consciously pay attention to the details, you would never accomplish anything.

You can use these principles to enliven the healing forces in your body, even though you may not have realized you can influence them. Awakening your inner healer requires a different set of procedures than the way you usually accomplish things. When you want to lift your hand, you send a signal from your brain to your spinal cord causing certain muscles to contract and others to relax. When you want to lower your blood pressure or improve your immune function, you must use a subtler approach that relies upon your attention and intention.

Try the following visualization and see if you are able to influence functions in your body that you may have previously not thought possible.

Healing Visualization

Sit quietly with your eyes closed for a few moments. Then bring your attention into your heart and acknowledge all the things for which you feel gratitude.

Now have the intention to release any grievance, regrets, or hostility you may be carrying in your heart or mind. Later, if you so choose, you can bring those grievances back into your consciousness. But for the time of this meditation let them go.

Now, for a moment or two, silently repeat the phrase *"Thy will be done."* Address this to your own vision of universal consciousness, whether you refer to it as God, or Spirit, or in any other way. Repeat *"Thy will be done,"* like a mantra.

Have the intention of quieting your internal dialogue—and allow your attention to move through your body. If you discover an area of tension, intend that it should be relaxed.

Next, bring your attention to your breathing. At first, just observe your breath—then intend for your breath to slow down.

Move awareness to your heart. Become aware of its beat, as sound and as feeling. Have an intention for your heart rate to slow down. Now bring attention to your hands. Feel the throbbing of your heartbeat in your hands. Feel the tingling and warmth that emanates from your heart. Intend to increase the blood flow and the temperature of your hands.

Move your awareness to your eyes. Feel the throbbing of your heartbeat in your eyes, and then in your face.

Now let your awareness move freely through your body. Feel the warmth, tingling, and throbbing of your heartbeat wherever you choose. If you find an area of your body that you believe needs healing, intend warmth for that area. If you are not aware of such an area in your body, just return awareness to your heart. But bring the throbbing warmth of your heartbeat to any point that you wish to nourish and heal.

Now, with awareness and intention of the healing area of your body, repeat for several minutes these two words, like a mantra: *healing and transformation.*

Move awareness back to your heart, without intention now. Just be aware of your heartbeat. Then move awareness to your breath. After a few moments, open your eyes to complete the healing meditation.

❖

This meditation first raises the temperature and blood flow to areas of the body that require nourishing attention, and then introduces the intention of healing. This is a very powerful meditation, and it's important to remember to go through the whole sequence, including the intentions of gratitude and relinquishing of grievances. Practice the healing meditation as often as possible. With time, you'll be able to experience warmth and tingling wherever you choose and be able to activate healing energy in your body through attention and intention.

MARMA THERAPY—STIMULATING THE POINTS WHERE MIND AND BODY MEET

Because there is intelligence in every cell, the mind and body meet everywhere, not just in the brain. In fact, once you strip off its physical mask, a cell is really a junction point between matter and consciousness, a station where the quantum mechanical body and the outside world intersect. Certain junction points are more vital than others, however. Ayurveda makes use of certain extremely sensitive points located on the skin. There are 107 of these *marmas*, as they are called. Though invisible to the eye, marmas are accessible through the sense of touch and are considered critical for maintaining balance throughout the body. A massage technique called marma therapy stimulates them; it is offered at our Center and once taught can be practiced at home.

Ancient Ayurvedic surgical texts warn the physician never to cut across the marmas, which have been mapped out precisely according to site and function. This is similar to but not exactly the same as the meridians mapped out by Chinese acupuncture; marma therapy predates the Chinese approach and is likely its direct ancestor. Avoiding damage to the marmas is a wise precaution. Although they do not usually intersect with prominent blood vessels or nerves, marmas are just as vital, since they mark out where the flow of inner intelligence is moving, indicating spots of maximum sensitivity and awareness.

STIMULATING THE MARMAS

By stimulating the marmas, the connection between consciousness and physiology can be enlivened. There are various ways to activate a marma. One is through the gentle yoga movements prescribed in part III under exercise. As you move your body in a yoga position, you are gently stretching specific marma points. The oil drip on the forehead used in panchakarma (called shirodhara) is profoundly soothing because the warm oil lands directly on a major marma point in the center of the forehead. Similarly, the daily oil massage (abhyanga) taught under daily routine reaches all the marmas on the skin. This contact is immediately registered throughout the nervous system. Marma points thus allow you to "talk" directly to Vata dosha and keep it in balance.

Since the marmas are not superficial but penetrate deep into the system, they can be stimulated mentally. Meditation enlivens all the marmas, but particularly the three "great marmas" (*Mahamarma*) situated in the area of the head, heart, and lower abdomen. These are not located on the surface of the skin and have to be stimulated by going directly to the quantum mechanical body; they are also the marmas you want to stimulate most, since they have a strong influence over the lesser marmas.

CLINICAL MARMA THERAPY

At the Chopra Center a special marma therapy is given that includes instruction for home treatment. Marma points are identified with each of the three doshas and stimulated with an appropriate essential oil mixture. A patient is first diagnosed according to specific imbalances. Let's say that a chronic headache has been associated with imbalance of Prana Vata, the subdosha of Vata located in the head. Trained technicians would gently massage in precise order those marma points that correspond to Prana Vata, applying prescribed herbalized oils. Patients find this treatment extremely relaxing, with some reporting alleviation of pain and other longstanding chronic symptoms.

MARMAS AT HOME

Since marmas have to be located with a trained eye, being slightly different from person to person, the clinical therapy cannot be taught in a book. You can take advantage of marmas in a more general way, however. A cluster of the most important points is located on the soles of the feet. To enliven them, a gentle foot massage with sesame oil lasting three to five minutes every day is recommended. A good time for this is at bedtime, because the soothing effect on the nervous system, and on Vata dosha in particular, makes this massage a good prelude to sleep.

Also, when you do your daily abhyanga, pay special attention to the three important marmas illustrated on page 181.

One is located between your eyebrows, extending to the center of the forehead. Gently massaging this area with eyes closed is good for worry, headaches, mental strain, and other upper Vata problems. The one connected to the heart (its actual location is just below the sternum, where the rib cage ends) is good for settling upset emotions. The one on the lower abdomen, about four inches below the navel, is good for constipation, gas, and other lower Vata problems. Use a light circular motion, taking a few minutes at each site. The forehead marma can be selected by itself as an aid to falling asleep at night, as long as you make sure that you never press hard or

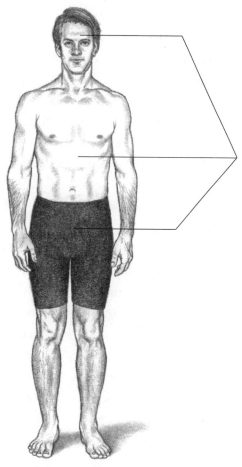

Three important marma points to massage at home.

rush—that would tend to disturb your Vata rather than inducing it to be more settled.

ACCESSING THE BLISS OF NATURE

If you think about an experience of joy—the birth of a child, the sight of a glorious sunset, or an alpine lake at dawn—and then carry your feelings beyond a fixed moment, you arrive at a new state called "pure joy." Ayurveda tells us that pure joy is a fundamental quality of life. In Sanskrit this quality is called *ananda*, which is usually translated as "bliss."

With the popularity of Eastern teachings in the West, people have come to use the word *bliss* to express many kinds of positive emotions. To be precise, bliss is too abstract to be experienced by itself. By analogy, how do you experience being intelligent? Like intelligence, bliss is an abstraction. It resides in the quantum mechanical body in pure form and bubbles to the surface only under the right conditions. You cannot see or touch the thousands of processes in brain and body that need to be coordinated in order to create bliss, but there is a definite feeling—pure joy—that can be felt and which proves that bliss exists.

According to the Ayurvedic sages, all of our joys stem from pure joy. It is the bright light we do not see directly but only by reflection in smaller joys. These lesser lights could not exist without the greater one. Even in Western society, where money, physical beauty, and success are equated with happiness, everyone has unexpected moments when life seems absolutely perfect and full of joy. If you could live in a state of pure joy all the time, you would have the practical essence of perfect health.

Tuning Into Nature's Gifts

Nature provides a rich source of energy and nourishment that has healing effects on both body and mind. Open yourself to the gifts of Nature through your five senses:

- Walk barefoot on the earth for a few minutes every day. Have your attention on your feet and the earth with the intention to absorb nourishment from the earth.
- Walk along natural bodies of water. Allow the cooling, coherent influence of water to infuse your being.

- Allow the light and warmth of the sun to permeate you. Acknowledge the energy-giving force of the sun, the source of all life on earth.
- Take a walk where there is abundant vegetation and deeply inhale the breath of plants. The ideal time to receive the life force of plants is right before dawn and right after sunset.
- Gaze into the stars at night. Allow your awareness to fill the heavens and the cosmos to fill your awareness.

THE NATURALNESS OF BLISS

Each dosha expresses a different flavor of joy, and in the state of perfect balance, one would be able to experience them all:

Vata—stimulating, exhilarating, alert, cheerful, optimistic, flexible

Pitta—content, joyous, chivalrous, pleasant, clear-minded

Kapha—steady, strong, forgiving, courageous, generous, affectionate, serene

As in most cases, Vata is the leader of the other doshas. It transmits joy through the nervous system, causing changes in cells throughout the body. But without balance among all three doshas, your physiology cannot support pure joy for extended periods. A major goal in Ayurveda is to change this by cleaning the windows of inner perception. Our normal waking-state perception of ourselves is usually ill-equipped to realize how much joy exists inside us.

Because conventional psychology concentrates so much on abnormal states, on neuroses and psychoses, it has had little to say about the effects of joy, and internal medicine has said nothing. Moments of ecstasy have certainly been prized—by poets, religious figures, and ordinary people—but the connection with higher states of health was not made until the psychologist Abraham Maslow, working in the 1950s and 1960s, began to study a group of high achievers whom he called "self-actualized." Such individuals, Maslow quickly discovered, led extremely diverse and highly individual lives. On the surface, there was no obvious resemblance between a successful entrepreneur, a famous novelist, and a great conductor. However, beneath their different lifestyles Maslow found that many had had what he termed "peak experiences," moments of intense well-being and joy.

During their peak moments, these people felt a total transformation of their personal reality. Obstacles that seemed huge in ordinary life became laughable. An overwhelming sense of power flooded through them. They felt deeply calm and in tune with life.

The most talented athletes and performers of all kinds will testify to moments when they effortlessly exceed their known skills. As women's basketball champion Patsy Neal describes it, "There are moments of glory that go beyond human expectation, beyond the physical and emotional ability of the individual. Something *unexplainable* takes over and breathes life into the known life. The athlete goes beyond herself; she transcends the natural—she almost *floats* through the performance, drawing on forces she has not previously been aware of."

A peak experience, Maslow found, was extremely therapeutic. His patients attributed major life changes to realizations that had suddenly come to them in peak moments: newfound confidence and creativity, unexpected solutions to baffling dilemmas, and a sureness that no fear could touch them. In some cases, long-standing depression and anxiety neuroses vanished overnight, never to return.

Maslow was tremendously impressed, and his pioneering study vastly extended the range of positive experiences that came to be considered normal for the human psyche. However, he did not find a way to give anyone a peak experience, nor did he find its source. Without a technique for transcending, he could only wait for those occasional moments when the curtains part and the psyche sees beyond its ordinary waking state.

SUPERFLUIDITY

Not long ago, clinical psychologists discovered an effortless state that creative people often fall into, popularly called "the flow." During periods of "flow," work projects seem to progress of their own accord, and even the deepest concentration requires no effort. As long as they are in the flow, creative people of all types feel a pleasurable sense of being lifted far above their ordinary capabilities. The drawback to the flow is that it cannot be taught to others or further developed in oneself. Fewer than 10 percent of ordinary people are said to experience it, and those who do are in the flow only intermittently. Still, this represented an advance over the minuscule group of self-realized people, which Maslow had estimated as less than one-tenth of 1 percent of the general population.

It was not until science began seriously to investigate meditation that the elusiveness of these phenomena was fully explained. It turns out that a peak experience or a sensation of being in the flow points to a deeper, more sustained state researchers have labeled "superfluidity." Superfluidity resembles the flow in that less effort is required in activity, but the effort is reduced to an absolute minimum. In the superfluid state, action becomes completely automatic—the doer merges into his task, the thinker into his thoughts, the artist into his art.

Here is a firsthand description from a meditator. "A soft but strong feeling of blissful evenness is present most of the time in both mind and body. Physically, it is experienced as an extremely delightful liveliness throughout the body. This evenness is so deep and stable that it is maintained in the face of great activity—it cushions one against all disruptions and makes all activity easy and enjoyable."

The term *superfluidity* comes from a class of peculiar materials called superfluids that were discovered in physics more than fifty years ago. When liquid helium, for example, is cooled so low that it approaches within a few degrees of absolute zero, −273 degrees C, it acquires the ability to flow up the sides of its container, to pass through holes almost infinitely small, and, if set in motion, to flow forever. The reason for this mystifying change in behavior is the cooling effect itself. At a low enough temperature, the helium atoms stop moving around in random fashion and instead become almost completely orderly, like an army that falls into parade-ground formation after milling around the field. Supercooled helium atoms are so orderly that they reach a frictionless state of superflow. A similar property of supercooled materials is superconductivity, the ability to conduct electricity without friction. Superconductivity also seems to defy normal laws of nature, but in fact it is a special property that arises quite naturally as long as certain special conditions are met.

In the same way, superfluidity in awareness appears when meditation "cools down" the thinking process. The mind discovers more orderliness at quieter levels of the thinking process until it nears the total orderliness of pure silence without slipping completely into it. At that exact point, the quantum boundary of the mind, it is still possible to think and act, but following different rules. One experiences effortless expansion and a kind of "friction-less" creativity that cannot be discovered in the ordinary waking state.

AROMATHERAPY—BALANCE THROUGH THE SENSE OF SMELL

Each of your five senses is formed by a different vibration in the quantum mechanical body. Vibrations of light falling on your retina cause a response that is quite distinct from the vibrations of touch that greet your fingers. This is how the "energy soup" of the universe gets sorted out into distinct sights, sounds, smells, and so on. The three doshas are also precisely tuned in to nature. Each one prefers to respond to one or more of the five senses:

Vata—hearing and touch
Pitta—sight
Kapha—taste and smell

These preferences can be seen very easily in people whose body types are dominated by one dosha. Pure Vatas are extremely sensitive to loud noise and have skin that feels the slightest touch. Pitta types, particularly if fair-haired and light-skinned, cannot bear bright sunlight for any length of time and are also very responsive to visual beauty. Kaphas, the earthiest of types, love the atmosphere of hearth and home; to them, the tastes and smells of the kitchen are especially gratifying.

Since we all possess Vata, Pitta, and Kapha, these preferences are relative. Any body type can respond to marma therapy, for example, which operates through the sense of touch; it is not restricted to Vatas alone. The ancient Ayurvedic texts provide us with long lists of sensory stimuli that help to balance the doshas, from looking at the full moon and walking by water (very good for Pitta), to listening to the wind in the trees (very good for Vata). Out of this knowledge, a special treatment called aromatherapy has been developed; our patients find it absolutely delightful to undergo.

THE VOCABULARY OF AROMAS

Each dosha can be balanced with aromas that are matched to it. The matching is done by the *rasas*, or tastes, found in food. I will have a lot to say about the rasas in part III under diet. For the moment, note that there are six tastes in Ayurveda, the usual four of sweet, sour, salty, and bitter, plus astringent (the dry, mouth-puckering taste associated with beans, pomegranate, and turmeric) and pungent (spicy). Sweet foods are held to balance both Vata and Pitta, as does the sweet smell of a rose. Sour tastes aggravate Pitta, and so do sour smells, along with bad smells in general. Moist, earthy smells increase Kapha. Bitter and astringent smells particularly aggravate Vata.

The language of taste is limited to sweet, sour, salty, bitter, astringent, and pungent. The nose, on the other hand, understands a vast vocabulary of smells, amounting to about ten thousand different odors if you have a well-trained beak. The odors that can be detected by the nose must first dissolve in the moisture of the nasal tissue and are then passed on by specialized olfactory cells straight to the hypothalamus in the brain. (These olfactory cells are in fact nerves, the only ones exposed to the air in the whole body, although they are protected by their thin covering of mucus. They are also the only nerves that regenerate, replacing themselves about once every three weeks.)

The fact that smells go straight to the hypothalamus is very significant, for this tiny organ is responsible for regulating dozens of bodily functions, including temperature, thirst, hunger, blood-sugar levels, growth, sleeping, waking, sexual arousal, and emotions such as anger and happiness. To smell anything is to send an immediate message to "the brain's brain," and from it to the whole body.

At the same time, the message of an odor goes to the brain's limbic system, which processes emotions, and to an area called the hippocampus, the part of the brain responsible for memory, which is why smells bring back past memories so vividly. Kitchen smells, flowers, and perfumes all trigger a sense of déjà vu. The gardens you once walked through have turned into you, thanks to the lingering impression of their fragrance on your brain.

USING AROMATHERAPY

In Ayurveda, aromas are used to send specific signals that balance the three doshas. Generally speaking:

Vata is balanced with a mixture of warm, sweet, sour aromas like basil, orange, rose geranium, clove, and other spices.

Pitta is balanced by a mixture of sweet, cool aromas like sandalwood, rose, mint, cinnamon, and jasmine.

Kapha, similar to Vata, is balanced by a mixture of warm aromas, but with spicier overtones, like juniper, eucalyptus, camphor, clove, and marjoram.

Place about ten drops of aromatic oil in hot water and fill the room with a light scent for a half-hour; you can extend this time as long as you want, however. (Special candle-powered aroma pots are available, but using a teacup and miniature coffee warmer is just as effective.) Bedtime is good for inhaling the aroma, since the various sights and sounds of the day tend to cover over smells and block their effects. The aroma helps many people fall asleep and can be left in the room all night.

There is also a medical side to aromatherapy. Patients who have been diagnosed with specific imbalances are given oils for the subdosha that has gone out of balance. It is actually possible to restore balance with aroma if you know what subdosha you want to balance and which aroma pacifies it.

Sometime in February, Betsy Allen picked up a bad chest cold that kept her in bed for a week and refused to go away. Even after she was up and around, a dry, hacking cough continued to plague her. It lingered a month, then two, and when it reached the third month without resolving itself, she came for Ayurvedic evaluation.

She was diagnosed as a Vata-Pitta type with a localized Vata imbalance in the lining of her lungs. This can be treated in several ways. Her physician chose aromatherapy, prescribing a specific Vata oil she was to inhale at night. Betsy went home, not knowing what to expect.

"I didn't wait until bedtime," she recalls, "because my curiosity got the better of me. I just boiled up a teacup of water, put in a few drops of this sweet-smelling oil, and leaned over to sniff. The reaction in my body was very dramatic and totally unexpected. It was as if every cell, starting at the top of my head down to my toes, suddenly sprang to life. I just stood there taking in deep breaths one after another—I couldn't get enough of that smell!

"That night I used the aroma in the proper way, lying down in bed, and the same exhilarating energy came back again. My mind said this was an outrageous result to be getting from a *smell*, but my body was convinced." Very soon Betsy stopped coughing and fell asleep more easily than she had in months.

Without accurate diagnosis, aromatherapy is very general: it may possibly placate a symptom or merely seem pleasantly relaxing. We have been surprised at times when migraine headache, back pain, skin rash, and insomnia that have resisted other treatments, often for long periods of time, have responded to aromas. This testifies to the truth of the Ayurvedic principle that anything can be used as medicine if you know the patient well enough.

This technique requires no instruction other than what aroma oil to use. For those who cannot come in for medical evaluation, it is only possible to follow your dominant dosha—generally the one you are trying to pacify. You can order Vata, Pitta, or Kapha oils from the Internet source given on page 378; aroma pots and diffusers are also available.

MUSIC THERAPY—MELODIES TO BALANCE NATURE

Even as a child you probably experienced the influence that music can have on your body and mind. The lullaby your mother sang to you at bedtime helped you fall asleep. Songs at summer camp connected you with traditions going back generations. Singing in the Christmas choir inspired you.

Ayurveda recognizes that music can be used therapeutically to balance body and mind. Patients in our Center spend time every day listening to melodies that balance their doshas. Music therapy can provide a sophisticated method for changing physiology. Music is more than "soothing" or "rousing." Why do we listen to it in the first place? For pleasure, of course, but all pleasures change the body in some way. Ordinarily we do not measure our blood pressure to see how Bach or Mozart might be affecting it, but if you wanted to lower your blood pressure, listening to soft, slow classical music is considered very good medicine.

MUSIC AS MEDICINE

The fact that music can be a therapy came home to me in New Delhi at a conference for doctors on the clinical uses of music. At one point, a woman Ayurvedic physician stood up and announced that rather than talking about it, she would demonstrate what music therapy was all about.

She asked us to listen for a few minutes while she sang some Vedic melodies that specifically balance Vata. We closed our eyes as her voice sounded with a pulsating, exotic refrain that was very beguiling. The singing doctor then asked us to take the pulse of the person sitting next to us. When we did, every person reported a marked decrease in pulse rate from the norm of seventy to eighty beats a minute. Then she sang a quicker melody based on a different raga, or sequence of tones. Again we listened for a few minutes and took the pulse of the person next to us. Uniformly, the pulse rate had jumped above the norm. In effect, our bodies were being manipulated by sound in the direction our doctor wanted. This basic technique, with dozens of variations keyed to different parts of the body, constitutes the medical knowledge of music therapy. What lies behind it is the concept of balanced sound, vibrations that settle the doshas.

As with tastes, colors, and smells, a dosha is balanced by certain tones and disturbed by others. Playing fast or slow, tuning the instruments sharp or flat, and devising intricate rhythmic patterns are all techniques for changing the listener's response. Vedic musical texts have specified which ragas are appropriate for morning, noon, evening, and other times of day. When Vata is aroused to a peak by the busyness of work at four o'clock in the afternoon, for example, music can begin the transition toward the more relaxed functioning of early evening. When properly played, certain melodies are said to have universal effects. Our bodies are responding with changes that mirror the varying rhythms of nature.

It is not just your pulse that calms down in the evening, after all; every plant and animal reacts according to its own evening cycles, too. Vedic music therapy embodies the fundamental vibrations that pulsate through nature at every moment.

USING MUSIC THERAPY

Music therapy forms a standard part of the programs at our Center. For home use, a set of tapes or compact discs can be ordered on the Internet (see p. 378) and played in segments throughout the day. If you are having difficulty getting energized in the morning, invigorating music can be played. If you are having trouble turning down your mental activity at night, soothing sounds can be helpful. We have found both classical

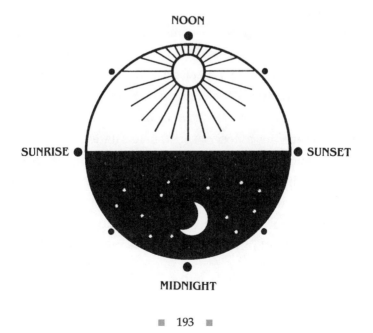

NOON

SUNRISE

SUNSET

MIDNIGHT

Indian music and contemporary adaptations to be very helpful in restoring mind body balance.

Just as the turning point from season to season makes your doshas especially vulnerable to imbalance (causing spring colds and late-summer allergies), your body is also sensitive to different times of the day. Bodily functions all have peaks at certain hours and troughs at others. Music therapy balances these into one continuous stream of rising and falling activity, eliminating extreme swings and rough transitions. If you try to go to sleep but can't because your mind is still racing with unfinished business from the day, you are witnessing the absence of a smooth transition. This is what music therapy can correct.

You can benefit from ten minutes of music therapy:

- As a gentle wakeup in the morning
- After a meal to settle digestion
- Just before bedtime as an aid to sleep
- During the recovery period when you are sick

The best way to listen is by sitting still with your eyes closed. Let your attention stay easily on the melody. If your mind wanders, bring it gently back to the music. When you are ready to get up, turn off the tape and sit for a minute or two in silence.

If you are trying to lose weight, listening to five minutes of Kapha balancing music several times daily will help increase your metabolism. If you are having trouble with irritability or heartburn, try listening to Pitta calming music. Whenever you are feeling anxious or worried, allowing your attention to stay easily and comfortably with Vata balancing music helps settle this turbulent dosha.

Find music that resonates with your nature. It can be classical Western music, traditional Indian ragas, Australian aboriginal rhythms, or contemporary instrumentals. Find the vibrations that are most nourishing to you and tune in to the effects the sounds have on your physiology. If you feel pleasantly refreshed, light, and alert, the music is working.

CHAPTER 8

FREEDOM FROM ADDICTIONS

Looked at starkly, our society is becoming more addicted every year. High-tech medicine, public campaigns to "Just Say No," and a multibillion-dollar rehabilitation industry have not solved this crushing social problem. For every encouraging trend, there seems to be a discouraging backlash. The overall rate of cigarette smoking has declined by about 15 percent from its height in 1960, but over 50 million Americans continue to smoke, and selected groups, especially teenage girls and working-class males, are smoking in record numbers. (As a result, female cases of lung cancer continue to rise.) It is estimated that 70 percent of cigarette smokers who begin as teenagers will continue smoking for forty years.

Alcohol consumption has switched from hard liquor to beer and wine, but alcoholism itself has filtered down to shockingly young ages; many junior high schools have been forced to run anti-alcohol campaigns. Alcohol and drug treatment programs exert mighty efforts to keep their participants free from addiction, but their success is limited. Hard drugs have proliferated alarmingly, and the connection between drugs and violent crime is at an all-time high. Again, young people are becoming involved—the sale of "crack" (smokable, synthetic cocaine) by school-age children is the latest, deeply troubling trend.

ROOTED IN MEMORY

The essence of quantum healing is that the memory of perfection cannot be lost, only covered over. Looking at someone who is addicted to alcohol, cigarettes, or drugs, it is apparent that a serious loss of balance is present, and that clear, healthy messages from the quantum mechanical body are either extremely distorted or nonexistent. What can Ayurveda do to improve this situation? First, we explain addictions in a new way, as a distortion of intelligence existing at a very deep level in the addict.

Instead of arguing over whether addiction is physical or mental, acquired or inherited, we point out that at the quantum level, all of these influences merge. What Ayurveda calls *smriti*, or memory, controls all the choices we make as biological organisms. In order for a cell to change, it must consult the blueprint inside itself where all its memories, functions, and tendencies are stored. If this blueprint is distorted, then a distorted cell will result.

❖

One of my most vivid memories is of Walter, a young black man who was raised in the slums of South Boston, mostly in the streets. He dropped out of school at 16 and joined the army the day he turned 18. Shipped to Vietnam, he saw active combat and emerged without being wounded, but when he returned home two years later, he was addicted to heroin, which many soldiers had used to make the war less traumatic. Unlike most soldiers, however, Walter did not have a good reason to kick his habit when he got home. Eventually the police caught up with him, and under court orders he became a patient at the local Veterans Administration hospital.

At the outset, the doctors' main concern with Walter was simply to detoxify him. Normally, he would have received little extra attention afterward. But while he was recovering, I began to visit him as a staff doctor at the facility. It was clear to me that Walter was an unusual case. Despite his desperate situation, Walter had retained hope and was courageously willing to fight his habit. He progressed rapidly under treatment, and a year after his detoxification he was holding down a steady job and talking eagerly about his future dreams and plans.

This future never materialized. One day Walter's car broke down, forcing him to take the subway to work, which he hadn't done in several months. He boarded a train to Dorchester, an antiquated line with decrepit, screeching equipment. Walter was bothered by the loud noise and couldn't manage to ignore it. It was a sweltering July day, and the fan was broken. Within a few minutes of being shut up in the stifling car, he found the train unbearable. In a matter of minutes he was extremely agitated, and by the time he got off, he was completely irrational. Nothing Walter did made his agitation subside. The next day, when he was brought back to the hospital, he was hooked on heroin worse than before. This time, he had no will to recover.

My notes read: "What happened to this man? A chemical explanation for the train incident is not sufficient. I keep thinking of him wearing his pinstriped business suit, confidently outfitted for a new life, but then having to step onto the train that he rode when he was troubled and addicted. In some treacherous twist of memory, the past came back, and with it came his craving. Where did the craving hide out for a year before it returned? The cells in everyone's body come and go, but their disappearance is not enough to break the spell that has the addict in its grip. In some way that medicine is just beginning to unravel, a cell's memory is able to outlive the cell itself."

If this is true, then one has to change the blueprint in memory to rid oneself of the addiction. It is not enough just to remove the physical toxins from the cells, to counsel the addicted person, or to try to teach him different behavior patterns. These steps are worth pursuing for their own sake, but the addiction is ultimately rooted in memory, and there is where it must be uprooted.

A HANDS-OFF CURE

As it stands now, typical programs for treating addicted people employ highly confrontational tactics, emphasizing the need for constant vigilance to guard against the possible return of the all-powerful habit. "The monkey is on your back," the addict is told, "and he'll be there for the rest of your life." The rationale for this insistence is that compulsive addicts will never be cured until they are turned into compulsive abstainers.

In Ayurveda our emphasis is exactly the opposite. The cornerstone of our addiction program is that the addict will give up his habit automatically when offered a greater source of satisfaction. We hold that the source of addiction is a search for satisfaction. Alcohol, cigarettes, and drugs cause untold damage, but their users derive some kind of pleasure from them, or at least relief from the massive stress that they would otherwise feel. Addicts maintain their habits for want of a way out. Bouts of guilt, shame, remorse, and self-accusation do very little to help.

But by exposing their minds to a greater source of satisfaction, the natural tendency would be to head away from the addiction, because the greater satisfaction is more appealing. Support for this new view has existed for almost twenty years. Going back many years, studies in the United States and Europe have repeatedly shown that when addicted people are taught to meditate, their level of anxiety decreases, pulling down with it their use of alcohol, cigarettes, and other drugs. If the addiction is caught at an early stage, a large proportion of subjects will stop abusing substances altogether. This is a very important point, because the early stage is where most cures are possible.

By removing the distractions of stress, meditation renews the nervous system's memory of balance. Repeated meditation, day after day, jogs the memory again and again, until in time the cells return to a normal state, exchanging their abnormal receptors for a more normal pattern. Once the pathways of intelligence are repaired, the cells will automatically select the body's healthy signals, as once they automatically accepted the distorted ones. The circle broken by addiction has been repaired.

The various studies on meditation and addiction have led to the following findings:

- In 1972, physiologist Robert Keith Wallace and coworkers surveyed 1,860 meditators, mainly college students, about their use of all kinds of drugs. After they began to meditate, the number of drug abusers dropped significantly in all categories (marijuana, narcotics, barbiturates, hallucinogens, and amphetamines). The longer the students practiced meditation, the less their dependence on drugs, until after twenty-one months, most had stopped abusing altogether. Marijuana was still used "very rarely" by 12 percent of the group; all other categories were in the range of 1 percent to 4 percent.

- A 1974 study on marijuana compared meditators with nonmeditators and found that after one to three months of meditation, about half of the meditators had decreased or stopped their use of the drug; by comparison, less than one-sixth of the nonmeditators had stopped using marijuana or decreased its use. These results improved dramatically the longer meditation continued. Among two-year meditators, 92 percent decreased their use of marijuana and 77 percent gave it up entirely. A similar study found the same results with alcohol.

- A high-school and college study asked 150 meditators and 110 controls about their drug history and found significant decreases in marijuana, wine, beer, and hard liquor in the meditators, while no decreases occurred among the nonmeditators.

All of these findings were based on people who had had no involvement in any sort of rehabilitation program. No one asked them to quit, followed their progress, or rewarded them for abstaining. Most important, no one was selected for having any motivation to abstain; indeed, in a college or high-school environment, the pressure comes in the opposite direction, from peers who abuse alcohol, cigarettes, and drugs. The decreases across the board suggest that simply by reducing stress and anxiety and raising the level of inner satisfaction, one can motivate addicts to stop their habits.

A stricter test of this principle occurs in institutions. A number of studies have focused on the use of meditation among prisoners, who have little or no motivation to quit their addictions. An overview of five such studies found that the results were significant enough to warrant placing meditation in prisons as a major treatment for drug abuse. A study in Germany looked at seventy-six drug abusers who enrolled in a drug rehabilitation program. After twelve months of meditating, decreases were found in all classes of drugs, including heroin, barbiturates, and amphetamines, which are among the hardest habits to kick.

By their very nature, statistical studies tend to be faceless. I like to return to individual stories, such as the one a veteran counselor in New York told me. He had been seeing a teenage girl who had started to drink before she was 12 and was severely alcoholic by the time she turned 15. She proved extremely resistant to all conventional rehabilitation, and in the end, after months of frustration, the counselor had to admit defeat. Just as he was releasing her from his program, he happened to remark, "Why don't you try meditating?" She showed some interest, but he was not able to follow up the case.

Some years later he noticed an attractive young mother in a local shopping center. With a start, he realized that it was the same girl, but now looking happy and even radiant walking her 2-year-old daughter. He went up to congratulate her.

"What happened to you?" he asked. As it turned out, she had begun meditation soon after dropping out of rehabilitation and stopped drinking on her own within a few months. She credited the meditation, which she still practiced, for saving her from deep addiction and probably for saving her life. The counselor has since then incorporated meditation into his work, starting many other addicts along the same road.

ADDICTION AND THE DOSHAS

All this indicates that there is a self-correcting mechanism inside the addict that can be triggered simply by allowing his mind to contact it. You can also see this mechanism at work in terms of the doshas. People who smoke or drink to excess, or who use drugs, have conditioned themselves away from the body's natural desire for balance. In the beginning, the ability to control their impulses may be fairly unimpaired; at this stage, addicted people believe that they are still in control of their habit.

Then ensues a period, lasting months or years, when all three doshas become chronically aggravated. Every addiction has its own profile of symptoms, but among chronic abusers we have always found that Pitta is grossly aggravated, giving rise to irrational moods of violence, flushed skin, abnormal sweating and thirst, and various digestive disorders, among other things.

Vata dosha seems particularly crucial, because its imbalance is responsible for impulsive behavior. When Vata is severely aggravated, any impulse to drink or to smoke a cigarette or to take a fix has to be obeyed. As impulse control starts to deteriorate, a huge amount of guilt is built up, since the addicted person identifies with his lack of control. Not knowing that he is following the command of Vata (as we all do, but in healthier forms), the addicted person sees only that his resolutions to quit are failing miserably.

In essence, Vata dosha itself is addicted. The stages of this addiction resemble those for any impairment of the central nervous system. That is why a hand tremor that is due to lack of sleep, Parkinson's disease, mental illness, or alcoholism all look basically the same to the untrained eye. Vata will generally go through the following stages of decline:

Mild imbalance: restless, scattered thoughts; increase of worries; easily startled; loss of memory and concentration; absence of inner freshness

Moderate imbalance: insomnia; loss of physical coordination; tremor in hands; anxiety, nervousness; loss of appetite; disconnected thinking; passing feelings of physical weakness and hollowness

Serious imbalance: chronic insomnia; impaired perception (things look distant and unreal); uncontrollable shaking of head and hands; no appetite; apathy, general loss of all desires; delusions and hallucinations

At the very end of an alcohol or drug addiction, Vata is often so out of control that the symptoms are practically indistinguishable from mental illness. A terminal alcoholic in the throes of DTs and a schizophrenic are both examples of Vata taken to its furthest limits.

The early and middle stages of addiction are the most treatable, because the body can be guided to rebalance itself. The catch-22 of all addictions is that the same symptoms of distress are caused by the habit and by stopping the habit. This makes perfect sense once you look at Vata dosha, which has become trained to accept the presence of the drug. As soon as the nicotine or alcohol is withdrawn, Vata tries to shake off its bad training and return to normal. When it heads back into balance, however, which requires throwing off excess Vata buildup, the body is more Vata than ever, hence the trembling, insomnia, and anxiety that accompany withdrawal.

When the nervous system has become chemically unbalanced, Vata has no anchor, no normal daily rhythm of rest and activity to stabilize the hundreds of other body rhythms that must be coordinated in a healthy person. Regular meditation provides the stability of deep rest alternating with activity. That is why people in the early stages of cigarette smoking and drug use find that they can drop their habits with no effort at all.

GIVING UP CIGARETTES

In the case of cigarette smoking, coaxing your body to give up its addiction makes much more sense than forcing it to. People do manage to quit by going "cold turkey," but the sudden withdrawal of nicotine precipitates a lot of stress. The story is told that Sigmund Freud smoked twenty cigars a day for many years, until he began to suffer heart palpitations as a result. He tried to quit smoking, on his doctor's advice, but the palpitations returned with doubled force as soon as he stopped, driving him back to his habit. Freud told his biographer that trying not to smoke was "torture beyond human power to bear."

In Ayurveda, we tell smokers to keep sending signals to the quantum mechanical body telling it that they want to quit. These signals can be of various kinds. Laying off cigarettes for a day at a time is one way—many if not most of the people who successfully quit do so by temporarily stopping a dozen or more times. A more powerful message is sent to the quantum mechanical body with meditation. Even if you are a heavy smoker, this may be all you need. One retrospective study based on five thousand meditators showed that only 1 percent of the men and 4 percent of the women were smokers, even though before starting meditators, a whopping 34 percent said that they smoked at least occasionally.

There are additional ways to help you quit. When patients come to Ayurveda clinics and ask how they can stop smoking as painlessly as possible, here is what we tell them. Three ground rules are laid down in advance:

1. Do not try to give up smoking—hard-minded determination just sets you up for failure. Nicotine is addictive, as is the habit of reaching for a cigarette. To end these

habits you have to retrain yourself as unconsciously as you started.

2. Keep your cigarettes with you—the strategy of throwing cigarettes away seems to make sense, but it only leads to panicked trips for more and the embarrassment of begging them from friends and strangers.

3. Notice the automatic cues that make you reach for a cigarette and dissociate yourself from them.

The third point is the key one and requires explanation. All smokers light up automatically on cue. For some the cue is picking up the phone, for others it is turning on the TV, starting a conversation, or ending a meal. You probably know your own cues; if not, take a day to observe them. These cues are the signals to Vata that make you act on impulse. You do not notice that you are lighting up because in fact your mind has gone blank for that instant. Vata has taken over.

You need to switch off this automatic pilot. The way to do that is surprisingly simple: smoke consciously and pay attention to the act of smoking. The best method, which has helped many of our patients to quit in a short period of time, is as follows:

- When you catch yourself lighting up, stop for a second and ask if you really want this cigarette.
- If so, go outside and sit quietly by yourself. Smoke the cigarette without distractions.
- As you are smoking, pay attention to your body. Feel the smoke in your lungs; feel any sensations in your mouth, nose, throat, stomach, or anywhere else.
- Take out a piece of paper or a small diary and immediately record what you felt and the time you smoked the

cigarette. Keep a record of each cigarette, whether it was conscious or automatic, and how it felt.

Do not worry about how much you are smoking; just record each cigarette, even if you find that at the end of a phone call you don't know how those three butts in the ashtray got there. If you follow this procedure faithfully, you will become a conscious smoker instead of a smoking machine. We have found that many patients cut down their daily intake from two packs to four or five cigarettes—this reflects how much they actually want to smoke. Cutting back is almost as important as stopping; it prepares the way for quitting and also reduces the direct health risk of your habit.

CURING AN ADDICTION AT HOME

In the past, many addicted people have preferred to live with their problem, no matter how tormenting, than to reveal it to outsiders. This feeling is entirely understandable, and I always feel it should be respected as long as you are also taking productive steps to quit. A complete course of home treatment would include:

- Learning to meditate
- Detoxifying the system, either at home or under a doctor's care
- Body-type diet (beginning with Vata-pacifying foods until the signs of Vata imbalance are gone)
- Regular Ayurvedic exercise
- Daily routine with oil massage (abhyanga) to settle disturbed Vata

At the outset, I recommend that you begin by learning to meditate at your local center, then visiting an Ayurvedic physician for a complete physical examination and diagnosis of imbalances. Tell him of your desire to quit, frankly and honestly. He will indicate how to detoxify your body and balance your doshas through diet and daily routine. Visiting him once a week thereafter is advisable at the outset, since the initial period is the most stressful for the body. But this is essentially a self-cure. Nobody coerces you into following the program; there is no confrontation or pressure of any kind.

Also be sure to take time every morning for a full-body abhyanga; a second, shorter massage at night, moving slowly and gently as you cover head, shoulders, and feet, is also recommended. And remember, the rule when you are quitting any habit is regularity. The more regular you can be about everything in your day, the better and quicker you will train Vata back to normal. You should not try to force Vata back into balance, since that is impossible; you want to coax and soothe it back. The gentlest time in your life should be the period when you are rebalancing your body.

In addition, a few other treatments enter into the picture as supplements:

- Music therapy
- Aromatherapy
- Herbal food supplements (known in Ayurveda as *rasayanas*—see page 221)

Listening to music is extremely settling to the nervous system while you are purifying your body. A fifteen-minute session in the morning is recommended, followed by another session at night before you go to bed. Filling your room with the appropriate dosha-pacifying aromas also helps relax you at bedtime. The use of rejuvenative herbal food supplements begins to repair the mind body connection at the level of your cells and strengthens tissues damaged by drugs.

We feel that no addiction treatment can succeed in the long run without compassion and understanding. If you decide to seek counseling, look for these qualities in a psychologist, pastor, doctor, or just a good friend. One crippling drawback of conventional rehabilitation is that constant vigilance means constant stress. The monkey never does get off your back. We feel instead that addicted people have to learn to trust themselves and be comfortable with their lifestyles. Any increase in fear and anxiety is totally unproductive, even if the stress is supposed to help end a habit. The rationale behind our hands-off approach is that nature can be trusted. An addict's body will return to balance if it is treated correctly.

If you are seriously addicted to alcohol or drugs, you may feel that you have ruined your whole life; most addicts have inflicted pain on their families and themselves. The vital thing for you to realize is that *this negativity is not you*. It is the result of physical and mental ama that has been built up over time. You should take the same attitude toward it that you would to dirt on your skin—wash it off and forget about it. If others want to remind you of how destructive you have been in the past, take their criticism as calmly as you can. The past is the past. You cannot live it over again, and you should not remind yourself of it.

It is extremely important that you associate with healthy, normal people as much as possible. You will have to choose whether to enroll in group rehabilitation—many addicted people feel that it is an important part of their return to normal life—but do everything you can to find a compassionate, positive counselor. Anyone who has a confrontational or fanatical approach to addictions should be avoided for your own good.

Finally, it is normal to have relapses as you are recovering. Of course you will be disappointed, but try to see that this is not a personal failure. It takes time for the body to normalize itself. If you have to have another drink, cigarette, or pill, it is the habituated doshas that are forcing you. Doshas are powerful, but you are much more powerful than they can ever be. Your essential self is untouched by addiction. It is happy, free, above all problems, and at peace. Once you begin to touch this true self of yours, everything will work out. Be patient and allow yourself to emerge in freedom.

The measure of your success is not how many days you go without a relapse. Rather, you should look for signs of self-acceptance; happiness, moments of joy and pleasure; return of a good appetite and love of food; better sleep, calmer dreams; lack of bad odors in the mouth and skin, less sweating; increased physical strength and endurance; and regular physical functioning (digestion, respiration, motor coordination, and so on).

All of these will come in time. The great joy of getting clean is that the body loves to be that way. I do not even favor the term *rehabilitation*. What you are doing is washing yourself off, inside and out. It is a natural process that will bring greater results the longer it continues. Temporary relapses are little more than minor obstacles, as long as you are willing to get back up and try again. A healthy, beautiful world is waiting for you and gets nearer with every step you take.

CHAPTER 9

AGING IS A MISTAKE

Although everyone falls prey to the aging process, no one has ever proved that it is necessary. One great advantage of the quantum mechanical body is that it does not age, a quality one sees throughout the quantum level of nature. Protons and neutrons do not grow older; nor does electricity or gravity. Life, which consists of these fundamental particles and forces, is astonishingly durable; your DNA has remained much the same for at least 600 million years. A horseshoe crab crawling in the muck of ancient seabeds bears no visible likeness to a dinosaur, or a dinosaur to a gorilla, but from the vantage point of DNA, these are tiny variations on one unending theme.

As far as its chemical bonds go, DNA is not glued together any more firmly than is a leaf or a speck of pollen. You would think that such a loosely gathered bundle of atoms would unravel over time, like an ancient, crumbling tapestry. Certainly the forces operating against DNA's survival are immense: physical wear and tear, random destructive mutations, invasion by competitive microbes, and above all entropy, the tendency of the physical universe to wind down like a neglected clock.

DNA has outlasted them all. Mountain ranges have been worn down to hills over the life span of DNA, and yet it is never worn down by even a thousandth of a millimeter. The glue of the quantum mechanical body is too strong. If DNA's inner intelligence is this powerful, defying time and the elements for aeons, it seems that aging is not natural at all. Ayurveda operates on this assumption. Looking past the fact that everyone ages, we go to the really important question, "Do we have to?" The ancient sages, renowned for their own immense longevity, ascribed aging to a "mistake of the intellect" (called *pragya aparadh* in Sanskrit).

This mistake consists of identifying oneself solely with the physical body. To extend life requires correcting the intellect's mistake, identifying with the quantum mechanical body instead. If you take your mind to a level of functioning that is beyond age, then your body will begin to be touched with the same quality. It will age more slowly because your mind tells it to, at the deepest level. Seeing yourself as free from aging, you in fact will be. This is a startlingly simple principle, as yet unrecognized in mainstream Western medicine, but as we will discover, it is valid.

AGING VERSUS HEALING

Aging seems so complicated that it is difficult even to pin down exactly what it is. A typical liver cell performs five hundred separate functions, which gives it five hundred different ways to go wrong. All of these possibilities constitute the ways in which it can age. On the other hand, the view that aging is complex may be wrong. Despite the thousand waves that bring it in, the ocean tide is a single phenomenon, driven by a single force. The same may be true of human aging, although we see it as hundreds of waves: disconnected aches and pains, new wrinkles around the eyes and deeper smile marks at the corner of the mouth, a slight but inexorable rise in blood pressure, a faint loss of hearing and eyesight, and innumerable other minor inconveniences.

Ayurveda tells us not to be fooled by this complex, distressing show. Aging is *only one thing*, the loss of intelligence. Healing, as we saw, is the ability of intelligence to repair itself. Aging is the opposite, gradually forgetting how to make things right after they go wrong.

Consider the cells of a newborn baby, which are fresh, full of vigor, unscarred by time. If you place them under a microscope side by side with old adult cells, there is a startling contrast. Old adult tissue is disturbingly ugly; its cells look battered and used up. It is, after all, a microscopic vision of an old body. It displays dark patches here and there where debris has collected and soft tissue has turned fibrous.

This drastic change appears to be the result of wear and tear, but DNA, which controls all the functions of cells, is virtually invulnerable to wear and tear, as we just observed. So we are led to conclude that some kind of invisible damage is at work. For example, an artery starts out in life looking perfectly smooth, shiny, and white, like a piece of rubber surgical tubing fresh from the factory. But this tubing is actually a community of cells that have gotten together and taken on the job of forming an artery, mastering the precise sequences needed. Before they joined at their specialized outpost, each cell could have wound up as part of the brain, the heart, or the stomach—every possibility was open, because every cell contains the same DNA.

Yet, evolution has dictated that these particular cells take up one job only, that of being an artery. However specialized, the job is not simple. Rubber tubing lies passively and lets liquid flow through it. Your arteries, on the other hand, respond to everything that happens to you, and their responses have to be both active and intelligent. In biology textbooks, we get the idea that a cell divides again and again until its time is up, after about fifty divisions, at which point it dies. But this is a drastically simplified, even a false view. A cell has experiences. It remembers what happens to it. It is capable of losing its skills if links in its innate knowledge are lost or damaged. By the same token, a cell could be new all the time, without decay, if it preserved its complete store of intelligence. The difference between life and death for a cell lies in its *smriti*, or memory. If you take the longest perspective, a perfect memory in a cell would lead to immortality, for there can be no death as long as renewal continues without flaws or mistakes.

Science has never proved that DNA is limited in its ability to run a cell in good working order. Each of your arteries contains the same DNA that formed the arteries in Stone Age humans fifty thousand years ago. If DNA can manage to make perfect arteries for five hundred centuries, each one containing millions of perfectly operating cells, there is no intrinsic reason why *your* DNA should botch the job after sixty years.

But the botching takes place, and in a lot fewer than sixty years. By age 12, a typical artery changes markedly in appearance. It begins to develop irregularities in the form of yellow fatty streaks. At the microscopic level, one finds that these irregularities started as a result of tiny, nearly invisible cracks on the inside of the arterial wall. A cell biologist can look at one cell from such an artery and see the indisputable signs of age. Over the next five decades, the signs become obvious even to a layman. If you were attending open-chest surgery and touched a piece of old aorta, the major artery leading from the heart, it would feel like a stiff pipe (often as stiff as bone, if arteriosclerosis has advanced far enough). Inside, it would be riddled with fatty pockets called plaque. You would have no

trouble seeing that a terrible mistake has been made somewhere.

How does one close the gap between one reality—the
immortality of DNA—and another—the frail life span of a
human being? In fact the two realities are very close. There is
no physical distance between us and our DNA. There is only a
gap that exists in the nonphysical realm of knowledge.

As I have made abundantly clear by now, Ayurveda makes
a shift away from the idea of the cell as a physical package of
molecules, adopting instead the idea of the cell as a package of
knowledge. As the illustration below indicates, knowledge is
dynamic. It is not packaged inertly, but in living form, as the
constant interplay of three elements.

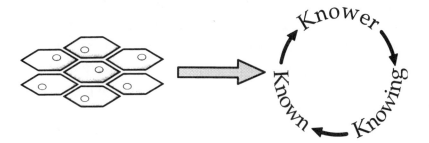

To have living knowledge, there must be a knower, an
object that it knows, and the process of knowing that connects
the two. The Vedic terms for this basic triad are *rishi* (knower),
devata (process of knowing), and *chhandas* (object of knowledge)—taken together, they form the totality of knowing, or
Samhita, the undivided state of pure awareness. The human
mind, then, is a three-in-one creation. A human body requires
the same simple ingredients, repeated countless times at different levels of the physiology. You are a knower, your body is
the object you form with your knowledge, and the millions of

cellular functions taking place inside you are the process of knowing. DNA too is a knower, but on a different scale, parceling out its knowledge in the form of biochemicals. On yet another scale, a red blood corpuscle is a knower, knowing how to attach itself to oxygen atoms for transport to all other cells in the body.

This threefold model of knowledge enables us to see how one thing—our inner intelligence—diversifies itself into endless combinations of things. Your 50 trillion cells, bound together as a community by hundreds of enzymes, proteins, peptides, amino acids, et cetera, represent an incredible display of one becoming many. Yet it is dangerous to get lost in the display. The "mistake of the intellect" occurs when the mind forgets its real source—the one intelligence flowing through every cell—and becomes hopelessly lost in the many. To prove that this is not just a philosophical point, let's turn to some groundbreaking experiments that demonstrate a startlingly simple solution to the aging process. To understand these experiments, we need a little background in physiology.

Chronological age (how old you are according to your birth certificate) is one way to measure the aging process, but not the most accurate one, since people vary widely in how their bodies change over time. Physiologists therefore refer to a second measure, called biological age, which measures the actual rate of aging in a person's cells, tissues, and organ systems. Chronological age matches biological age only when you are young. Two healthy 20-year-olds are likely to look almost identical if you compare their hearts, livers, skin, eyesight, and so on. But after middle age no two people have aged the same. Two 70-year-olds present drastically different profiles: one has arthritis, the other heart disease; one is myopic, the other not; and so on. This means that biological aging, though an accurate measure theoretically, is difficult to pin down, short of looking at every organ in the body. Fortunately, there are accepted ways to measure biological age, which include such things as near-point vision, acuity of hearing, and systolic blood pressure (the pressure in the blood vessels when the heart is pumping). These biological markers of aging usually deteriorate steadily over time; therefore, they give a reliable approximation of the biological age of the whole body at a given chronological age.

Several years ago a team of researchers made the exciting discovery that the biological markers of aging can be retarded or even reversed through meditation. The research was headed by Dr. R. Keith Wallace, a physiologist who studied eighty-four meditators with an average chronological age of 53. He divided his subjects into two groups according to how long they had been regularly practicing meditation. One group had meditated for at least five years, the other for fewer than five years.

Wallace found that meditation made his subjects biologically younger than their years, and by a considerable amount: the short-term meditators were five years younger than their chronological age, the long-term meditators a full twelve years younger. In other words, a woman of 60 who had been practicing meditation for at least five years would typically have the body of a 48-year-old, biologically speaking. (This does not include cosmetic changes in skin and hair, although many of the subjects did have strikingly youthful appearances.) These results did not depend on any other factor; people were screened for diet, exercise, and other habits. Interestingly, the controls revealed that not eating red meat was correlated with a slightly younger biological age, in keeping with various findings on the longer life span of vegetarians.

Wallace's findings were unprecedented at the time. Follow-up studies were soon conducted in England that confirmed his research. In one group, meditators were seven years younger in their biological age. When the same people were measured a year and a half later, they scored a further drop of one and a half years, implying that a year of meditation takes off a year of biological age.

More recently, Dr. Jay Glaser, a physician with a strong background in meditation, decided to pursue one of the naturally occurring chemicals in our bodies that may be connected with longevity. He measured the level of an adrenal hormone called DHEA (dehydroepiandrosterone) in meditators. Although the precise function of this hormone remains mysterious, it is known that DHEA reaches its highest levels at around age 25 and then declines in almost a straight line, year by year, until by age 70 only 5 percent of it remains. Initial enthusiasm over DHEA developed when it was injected in large doses into laboratory animals and showed striking anti-aging properties. Older animals showed renewed vigor, improved immunity, increased muscle tone, and better memory.

Glaser found that levels of DHEA were significantly higher in all ages of meditators compared to a matched group of nonmeditators. This was true for both men and women, with the biggest difference showing up in the oldest subjects. For example, Glaser found that the older meditators had the same DHEA as nonmeditators five to ten years younger. He interpreted these finding to suggest that meditation somehow increases the natural production of this interesting hormone.

Researchers have studied the effects of giving DHEA to people with mixed results. Although experiments with DHEA have shown that it causes changes in hormonal levels and may improve people's mood, it has not yet been found to have the same convincing benefits on memory or vitality in humans as it does in animals. Still, it is intriguing that a simple mental meditation technique can induce changes in a hormone that seems to play a role in the aging process. This biochemical clue gives support to the experience of people meditating who often report that they feel mentally and physically younger.

RASAYANAS—HERBS FOR LONGEVITY

Herbs are an immense part of Ayurvedic medicine that we have not yet touched on. Many thousands of medicinal herbs are prescribed in Ayurveda, and experienced Ayurvedic doctors often include herbs as part of their treatment. This is because herbs are not the same as drugs, but are more general and milder in effect. The simplest way to view herbs is as concentrated food. One of the ways in which herbs are traditionally classified is according to taste, using the six rasas—sweet, sour, salty, bitter, pungent, and astringent—that apply to food.

However, herbs are more potent and specific in their action. A bitter herb like quinine can bring Pitta down promptly, making it useful for reducing fever and inflammation. A pungent chili can instantly drain excess mucus as it reduces Kapha. An astringent spice like turmeric can dry the phlegm in a sore throat in a matter of minutes. In the section on diet in part III, I give some of the common household herbs that can be used at home to balance your doshas. Using herbs in combination with food is a safe approach.

For treating disease, stronger herbs are employed, which need to be medically supervised. In our Center we use specific herbs in the context of a holistic approach. Ayurvedic herbs are usually taken from the whole plant, which reduces the possibility of harmful side effects. The principle here is that the herb's active ingredient is packaged in the plant with other chemicals that buffer it, offsetting its possible undesirable actions. In other words, in Ayurveda the whole plant is part of nature's pharmacy. In Western medicine, however, only the active ingredient is regarded as useful.

How Ayurvedic Herbs Work

As they apply to longevity, the Ayurvedic texts list some special herbs, alone or in combination, that are classified as *rasayana*. The word loosely translates as "nourishing the essence of life." Rasayanas are not youth potions, they are correctives for loss of memory in the cells. Each herb is a packet of vibrations that specifically matches a vibration in the quantum mechanical body.

The liver, for example, is built up from a specific sequence of vibrations at the quantum level. In the case of liver malfunction, some disruption of the proper sequence in these vibrations is at fault. According to Ayurveda, an herb exists with this exact same sequence, and when applied, it restores the liver's functioning.

The principle at work here is called *complementarity*. Complementarity holds that "nature thinks everywhere alike," a Vedic slogan that means that nature uses the same materials when making plants, minerals, mantras, or human bodies. These are not just similar molecules (although it is the same carbon that goes into coal, diamonds, sugar, and blood). What is more basic still are the subtle vibrations that hold molecules together; these are the real building blocks of nature, according to the Vedic sages. They are so universal that seemingly unrelated things, such as a Sanskrit word and a bay leaf, can be considered kindred, if you know how to look deep enough. Because there is likeness everywhere in nature, an Ayurvedic doctor looks upon herbs, primordial sounds, gemstones, colors, aromas, and foods as equally fit to act as medicine. As used in Ayurveda, herbs do not have the same effect on the body that Western medicines do. Our drugs kill pain, relax muscles, replace deficient insulin or thyroid hormone, and so on; rasayanas introduce a subtle signal into the physiology—they "talk" to the doshas and directly influence the flow of inner intelligence.

Rasayanas are closely associated with Indian food and therefore are sold in the United States as herbal food supplements, not medicine. Some sweet fruits, such as Indian gooseberry (called *amla* or *amalaki*), are considered extremely good rasayanas. (In fact, this particular fruit forms the basis of most of the health tonics that have been taken since ancestral times in India as ginseng is taken in China.) To anyone interested in medicinal herbs, the lore of rasayana is fascinating, but also extremely complex. Dozens of plants are said to be capable of rejuvenating the body. Among those that have common names in Western herbalism:

- Gotu kola and garlic are specifics for Vata
- Aloe vera and saffron are specifics for Pitta
- Elecampane and honey are specifics for Kapha (although not an herb, honey is considered the *shukra*, or purest essence, of the plant world).

But this list does not include the most powerful rasayanas, which only have Indian names, among them *amla*, *guggul*, *shatavari*, and *ashwaghanda*.

What makes rasayanas complex is not just their reliance on fruits and herbs. To extract the desired effect from an ingredient, one must know when to pick it, how long to cook it and by what method, and in what proportion to blend it with other herbs. The recipe for a single rasayana may call for fifty ingredients, each of which must be carefully blended.

HERBAL REJUVENATIVES

After several years of investigation and trial, we feel that rasayana is a valuable field. It has yielded a few authentic formulas that have been re-created from the ancient recipes. Although rasayanas have been used for thousands of years by Ayurvedic physicians to enhance energy and immunity, we are only beginning to scientifically research the purported health benefits of these herbal compounds. Regulations governing herbs in this country permit the distribution of rasayanas as an adjunct to diet only; as such we recommend them for general use. No health claims are made for them nor are they to be used as medicine. (If you have been diagnosed with a specific illness, please do not take these or any other herbs without first consulting a physician trained in Ayurveda.)

Among the best known rasayanas is *Chavanprash*, based upon the fruit Indian gooseberry. This fruit, which is one of the highest natural sources of vitamin C, is known as *Amla* or *Dhatri* in Sanskrit, which means having the healing qualities of a nurse or mother. It has been classically used as a rejuvenative for the blood, heart, lungs, and reproductive tissues. We have formulated a modern version of Chavanprash known as *Biochavan*.

Another important classical Ayurvedic rasayana is *Brahmi Rasayana*, based upon the herb gotu kola. It is traditionally used as a revitalizer for the brain and nervous system. It is said to both calm restlessness and enhance awareness.

Intrigued by the vast classical Ayurvedic literature on rasayanas, researchers have undertaken studies in this country and Europe to determine what pharmacological actions these preparations have. The ingredients in these rasayanas seem to have potent antioxidant effects and may also inhibit the blood clotting cascade that is associated with the release of stress hormones.

Although it is clearly too early to extrapolate these studies on animals to humans, it is encouraging that these ancient natural herbal compounds are now receiving serious scientific attention. Ongoing research should help to clarify the role that these formulas can play in maintaining health and reversing disease.

The explanations offered for the potential benefits suggested by preliminary studies point to the possible role of free radical chemicals in a wide range of diseases. Free radicals are undesirable peroxides that have long been implicated in hastening the aging process; one of the main reasons for the popularity of vitamins E, C, and beta-carotene as anti-aging supplements is their ability to attach to free radicals and scavenge them before they can do harm to living tissues. Hopefully further understanding the mechanism and action of rasayanas will help substantiate the ancient claims of the benefits of these natural tonics to enhance vitality throughout one's life span.

At the Chopra Center for Well Being in La Jolla, California, we have been using rasayana preparations to enhance energy and vitality in our patients. We have separate formulations for men and women and are encouraged by the subjective reports of our patients. Further information on how to access these formulations is provided in Appendix A.

QUIZ: HOW WELL AM I AGING?

There is no separate "life extension" program in Ayurveda, for the simple reason that all of its approaches—diet, exercise, daily and seasonal routines, meditation, and the various healing techniques—are meant to enhance longevity. Considering the superior health of our patients today, we have every hope that a breakthrough in aging has been made. The classic Ayurvedic texts define one hundred years as a normal life span without infirmity or disease. We are aiming for at least that.

Can you prove to yourself that you are getting younger by following this program? Simple as it sounds, feeling happy and healthy is one good yardstick; being young at heart is recognized as a marker of long life. On a more objective basis, researchers at Duke University have compiled a short list of health factors correlated with longevity. Statistically speaking, people who rate well on each of these points have the best chance of living longer than average.

The following quiz is based on the Duke inventory. The most precise way to use it is in conjunction with a complete physical examination, but an informal personal rating will still tell you a lot. Being as honest and objective as you can, answer every question, giving yourself:

10 points for Excellent
5 points for Average
0 points for Below Average

Having arrived at a final score, follow Ayurveda for six months, then rate yourself again. The chances are very good that you will notice a surprisingly large improvement, and it is likely to occur well before the six months are up.

The following factors are listed in order of relative importance:

A. CARDIOVASCULAR DISEASE:

How many of your parents and grandparents suffered a premature heart attack or stroke (before age 60)?

None	10 points	
One or two	5 points	
Three or more	0 points	_____

My last cholesterol reading was

Excellent (Under 200 mg.)	10 points	
Average (220 mg.)	5 points	
Poor (over 240 mg.)	0 points	_____

My last blood pressure reading was

Excellent (120/70)	10 points	
Fair (130/90)	5 points	
Poor (140/95 or higher)	0 points	_____

(To be accurate, blood pressure should be measured three times, at different periods of the day.)

B. JOB SATISFACTION:

When I go to work in the morning, I feel

Eager for new challenges	10 points	
Ready to do the job, but not excited	5 points	
Uninterested—it's only a job	0 points	_____

C. CIGARETTE SMOKING:

Over the last five years I have

Never smoked	10 points	
Smoked occasionally	5 points	
Smoked regularly	0 points	_____

D. PHYSICAL FUNCTION:

This category includes a wide variety of indicators, such as physical coordination, efficient breathing, fast reaction time, good circulation, et cetera. To rate yourself, compare your physical fitness today with how your body performed ten years ago.

I feel almost exactly the same	10 points	
I notice a few things wrong	5 points	
I have a medical condition under treatment	0 points	_____

E. HAPPINESS:

All things considered, my life these days has been

Very fortunate	10 points	
Pretty good most of the time	5 points	
About as good as the next person's	0 points	_____

F. SELF-HEALTH RATING:

This year my general health has been

Excellent	10 points	
Good	5 points	
Fair or poor	0 points	_____

G. GENERAL INTELLIGENCE:

On IQ tests I come out

Above average (120 and over)	10 points	
Average (100–110)	5 points	
Below average (90 or below)	0 points	_____

FINAL SCORE _____

To rate yourself: A perfect score (90 points) indicates that you are very likely to live longer, perhaps much longer, than the national average (roughly age 78 for women and 72 for men). An above-average score (between 65 and 90) suggests that your life expectancy will be at least three years higher than the national norm, more if you are already past middle age. An average score (45–65) indicates an average life expectancy. A below-average score (below 40) indicates that you need to pay more attention to your health. It is not a cause for panic, because following the programs of Ayurveda should lead to noticeable improvements very quickly.

To gain a more accurate idea of where you stand, you can refine your score by considering a few other factors:

Age: High scores mean more as you get older. If you are over 50, a score in the 75–90 range indicates an enhanced likelihood of long life; the same score would not be as significant if you are only 30.

Lifestyle habits: All things being equal, regular habits are correlated with long life; these include eating three meals a day, getting eight hours of sleep each night, going to bed on time, and so on. Also, being married is indicative of a longer life expectancy than being single. Alcohol consumption should be minimal or none; alcoholism is known to reduce life expectancy.

Weight: Maintaining an ideal weight is best, although there is no harm in being ten to fifteen pounds overweight. Life span is shortened if you are obese (15 percent or more over your ideal weight) or if your weight has fluctuated drastically over a period of years.

How to Improve Your Score

As a result of the extensive research done on meditation, we can validate that our Ayurvedic program may improve each of the Duke University longevity factors. If we place the results in the context of Ayurveda as a whole, they become even stronger.

- Research with rasayanas suggests that they may offset several deleterious aspects of the aging process, including a beneficial effect on blood clotting, and a reduced susceptibility to carcinogens. Preliminary studies suggest that rasayanas may be effective as free radical scavengers that would positively impact the aging process.
- A pilot study on the effects of panchakarma suggests that this purification procedure enhances the rejuvenating

effect of meditation (ten meditating subjects became on average six years younger biologically over the period of a year while taking regular panchakarma, as opposed to one and a half years with meditation alone).

What all of this implies is that a complete Ayurvedic program should be even more effective than meditation by itself, and in fact may lead to all the powerful rejuvenating effects promised in the ancient texts. A basic program would include meditation, the appropriate Ayurvedic body-type diet, supplemented with rasayanas, regular exercise, panchakarma treatment at least once a year, and the major points given in the daily routine, or *dinacharya*, to be discussed in chapter 11.

PART III

LIVING IN TUNE WITH NATURE

CHAPTER 10

THE IMPULSE TO EVOLVE

The phrase "living in tune with nature" means something very precise in Ayurveda: having healthy desires that match what you actually need. As nature made you, what you need and what you want should not conflict. This is because all desires originate at the quantum level, as faint vibrations whose dynamic interaction is always balanced. If either the body or the mind tip out of balance, a correcting impulse is sent from the quantum body, and you register it as something you desire.

At this moment, millions of impulses are flowing through your nervous system, turning into all the actions you perform every day. To want a drink of water, for example, satisfies the separate need of 50 trillion cells in your body, each of which sends a message to be decoded by special receptors in the hypothalamus. In turn, the hypothalamus makes the mind body connection by manufacturing the specific neurotransmitters, or messenger molecules, that make you think, "I'm thirsty."

A natural desire of any kind takes a similar path. A need arises somewhere in the quantum mechanical body, the mind body connection is made in the brain, and then you experience an impulse to act. As long as needs and desires match, you are living in tune with nature; the path of desire is not blocked. Ideally, every bite of food you eat should taste delicious to you and at the same time satisfy a precise demand for nutrients. Your skin may be asking for extra vitamin C to repair damage from a sunburn, a stressed hipbone may be asking for extra calcium, a flexed arm muscle for more potassium.

Unfortunately, it is very easy to interfere with this pathway, and when we do so, we slip out of tune with nature. Instead of trusting the balanced body to tell us what nutrients it needs, all too often we indiscriminately take vitamins, compulsively overeat, crave far too many sweets and junk foods of all kinds. The current vogue of "life extension" is based on distrust of the body, trying to second-guess its weaknesses by cramming it with megadoses of vitamin E, beta-carotene, selenium, or whatever new nutriceutical has joined the list.

It has not been proved that taking supplementary vitamins and minerals alone prolongs life. On the contrary, separate studies conducted in Southern California showed that older people who obsessively take vitamins and eat only "health food" do not live any longer than average, while people who have balanced lifestyle habits (going to bed on time, eating three meals a day, drinking alcohol only very moderately, and so on) live up to eleven years longer than the norm.

You do not have to go to an extreme to get the most from your body. The body is intelligent. At the quantum level, it knows exactly what it needs, down to the last atom and molecule of food, the faintest breath you breathe, the smallest action you take. In the following chapters, I outline the kind of foods, exercise, and daily and seasonal routines that Ayurveda considers in tune with nature. Although very specific, these guidelines are not rules but pointers to put you in touch with your quantum mechanical body. Once you are back in touch, action goes much more smoothly, correct choices become more automatic, and mistakes become less frequent.

Before getting into specifics, though, I'd like to say more about the evolutionary path itself.

MAKING RIGHT CHOICES

To continue evolving and progressing in life, you must make the right choices for yourself, day after day, minute after minute. The choices are endless because the challenges of life are endless, so to avoid all the wrong choices seems imposs-ible. But Ayurveda says that in fact it is easy—once you begin to listen to your own deepest nature.

For every decision you make, major or mundane, your quantum mechanical body sees only one correct choice, although your mind might recognize many. This confusion gives rise to internal conflict. Why does a smoker compul-sively reach for another cigarette, knowing the harm it can do? Why does a compulsive eater take second helpings in the absence of hunger? Wrestling with these conflicts is futile— our actions are based on too many individual processes, all of them changing all the time. Defeating lethal viruses or bacteria is child's play compared with trying to defeat people's self-destructive habits. For example, we all know chronically over-weight people who have turned everywhere for a cure, to drugs, psychiatry, behavior modification, and even surgery, with little or no success.

In Ayurveda we propose a simpler solution. Instead of wrestling with all the wrong choices people are likely to make in the grip of unhealthy desires, we put our patients in touch with the source of their desires. At the source, everyone has healthy desires. In Sanskrit, this is called *sattva*, a word often translated as "purity." A better translation of sattva is "the impulse to evolve," and I will demonstrate why.

In Ayurveda there are three natural impulses at work in any given situation. One is sattva, the impulse to evolve, to go forward, to progress. The second impulse is *tamas*, the exact opposite, the impulse to stay the same or to regress. Fixed between these two opposites is *rajas*, a more neutral impulse that dictates action for its own sake. A diagram of the three looks like this:

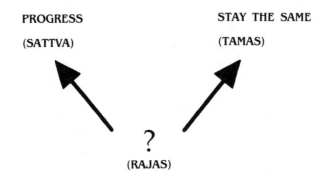

PROGRESS

(SATTVA)

STAY THE SAME

(TAMAS)

?

(RAJAS)

As you can see, rajas poses the question, "How should I act in this situation?" Sattva favors the choice that is evolutionary, tamas the one that is stable. All three impulses are necessary to life. If you are sitting up late at night, tempted to watch the second late movie on TV, one impulse tells you to go to bed, while its opposite tells you to continue sitting there. This is sattva and tamas in conflict, with rajas acting as the spur, urging you to choose.

Nature has made us so that our minds instinctively operate according to these three gunas, or tendencies (they are also sometimes called "the mental doshas"). People can be classified according to which of these three gunas is generally dominant.

Rajasic people like to act. Their minds work constantly and tend toward impatience, impulsiveness, and kinetic outlets of all kinds.

Sattvic people like to progress. Their minds do not dwell on action for its own sake, but only on action that is creative, life-supporting, and healthy.

Tamasic people like to stay the same. Their minds do not like to act; they enjoy set routines and tend toward the status quo.

These types are not cut and dried, since everyone contains elements of each. But all of us know pure rajasic types— extroverted, endlessly full of energy, people who rush in where angels fear to tread. And we know pure tamasic types—slow to move, resistant to new ideas, hard-core traditionalists for whom the best things in life are always in the past. (Ayurvedic doctors who come to America from India often shake their heads and say that we are a hopelessly rajasic people, whose creativity and ambition need more of the gentle, purifying element of sattva.) However we were shaped by nature, becoming more sattvic is a worthwhile goal, for it is sattva that makes a person more creative, healthier, and happier.

The secret of sattvic people is that they have naturally healthy desires. Unhealthy desires can arise in anyone because of mental ama. You will remember that "mental ama" is the term used for impurities, or negative tendencies in the mind. Sattva is the force of purity that combats them. The Ayurvedic sages say that mental ama is produced by:

- Negative emotions—anger, fear, self-criticism, greed, resentment

- Psychological stress—family problems, tensions at work, loss of money or job, divorce, death in the family
- Lethargy, mental inertia
- Unwholesome surroundings
- Contact with other people's negativity
- Violent, crude, or shocking books or other forms of entertainment

The debate over whether it is morally right to show violence on television misses the essential point, according to Ayurveda. The issue is one of health. The sight of violence gets translated into unhealthy chemicals in the body, leading to the buildup of ama in our thoughts as well as in our cells. Everyone has a right to expose himself to any kind of influence he wants, but the physician's role is to warn against those influences that damage our well-being. Avoiding mental ama is therefore considered a preventive measure against the imbalances that lead ultimately to disease.

You cannot force your body to make evolutionary choices. If you are eating the wrong foods, chain-smoking, drinking excessively, or making any other kind of unhealthy choice in your daily life, some block exists somewhere in your pathway of desire. Some impurity is keeping you away from your quantum self. I have already given many techniques for removing such blockages. All of these, from panchakarma to meditation to the bliss technique, remove tremendous amounts of impurity every time you use them.

After a while, as you continue using the Ayurvedic techniques, you will see your sattvic side emerge, no matter how blocked your system was to begin with. When that happens, you are approaching the place called perfect health. Sattva lies closest to nature's heart, because everything in nature expands, evolves, and grows. Sattva exists in us as our instinct for balance, our life-enhancing attitudes, our innate dignity and respect for others, and our love. As you increase in sattva, you effortlessly live in purity and move in the direction of higher evolution. Then and only then does the phrase "living in tune with nature" reveal its real meaning.

HOW TO INCREASE SATTVA

Ayurveda says that many different kinds of influences can increase sattva, while at the same time keeping ama at a minimum. Some recommendations are familiar to us: consuming pure food and water, avoiding obvious toxins such as pesticides, and getting a full night's sleep. Adequate rest is needed to bring out the clear, happy side of the mind.

Spend time outside in nature, walking in the woods and mountains or beside the ocean, lakes, and streams; listen to the sound of the wind, the rustling of the trees, and the songs of birds—all of these purify the senses and bring them back to their source in nature. In Ayurveda we consider anything that is life-supporting to be sattvic, so nurturing positive emotions and secure relationships is vital—the absence of love and care from your life will damage sattva far more than any wrong diet.

In addition, the following pointers, established thousands of years ago in the Vedic texts and echoed in the purest traditions of every culture, serve as time-tested guides for increasing sattva in daily life:

- Be pleasant and tolerant toward everyone.
- Act on due reflection, not on impulse.
- Refrain from anger or criticism, even when you feel it is justified (sattvic people do not point out others' weaknesses "for their own good").

- Take time every day for play, humor, relaxation, and good company.
- Wake with the sun in the morning, watch the sun set in the evening, and occasionally stroll in the moonlight, especially if there is a full moon.
- Eat light, natural foods, favoring milk, saffron, rice, and ghee (clarified butter)—a complete list of sattvic foods is given on page 307, along with the deeper rationale for adhering to a pure diet.
- Be generous with others in every way—giving presents and compliments to people around you, pointing out the best in everyone, letting others make you great instead of trying to be great yourself. To a sattvic person, all relationships exist primarily as an opportunity to give. The complement to this basic attitude is that nature will always provide enough to fulfill one's needs. When this kind of generosity and trust truly blossoms, a sattvic person has nothing to fear from life and everything to receive from it; he can let life happen without forcing it.

CHAPTER 11

DAILY ROUTINE—RIDING NATURE'S WAVES

Every day the sun rises, the sun sets, and hundreds of different things happen in between. Nature is so beautifully arranged that no matter how different these things are, they fit into one rhythm. Actually, there are many rhythms nestled inside one another, wheels within wheels. Modern medicine has disclosed many of the more obvious cycles in our bodies—the heart beating every three-quarters of a second, the lungs swelling to inhale air ten to fourteen times a minute. But many of the body's changes remain mysterious. Why does a person typically weigh the most at seven in the evening, as science has discovered? Why are our hands hottest at around two in the morning?

Ayurveda's answer is that there are "master cycles" in us governed by the quantum mechanical body. Every day two waves of change pass through us, each bringing a Kapha cycle, then a Pitta, and finally a Vata cycle. These three phases take place from sunrise to sunset, then again from sunset to sunrise. The approximate times are as follows:

FIRST CYCLE   SECOND CYCLE

6 A.M. to 10 A.M.—Kapha   6 P.M. to 10 P.M.—Kapha

10 A.M. to 2 P.M.—Pitta   10 P.M. to 2 A.M.—Pitta

2 P.M. to 6 P.M.—Vata   2 A.M. to 6 A.M.—Vata

One of the most basic aspects of living in tune with nature is to respect these master cycles that support our physical existence. We are meant to ride nature's waves, not to fight against them. In fact, our bodies are already riding them, or doing the best they can in the face of our contrary habits.

At dawn, the day begins in a Kapha period. It is easy to see why early morning is considered Kapha—waking up, the body feels slow, heavy, relaxed, and calm, all of which are Kapha qualities. The most physically active time and also the peak of appetite occur at noon, in the middle of the first Pitta period. Pitta is responsible for metabolizing food, for distributing energy, and for more efficient physical functioning in general. This helps explain why factory work reaches a peak of efficiency at noon. This first cycle ends with a Vata period beginning at 2 P.M. Vata controls the nervous system, and in fact researchers have discovered that people do best in mental tests during the afternoon. The times when you can add numbers the fastest (3 P.M.) and exhibit the most manual dexterity (4 P.M.) fall into this Vata period.

The day's second cycle repeats the same sequence of Kapha, Pitta, and Vata, but they take on a different complexion. The evening is relaxed and slow, just like the early morning, but sunset brings the body back to a stable resting place. Now Kapha inclines toward inertia. Similarly, Pitta appetite is not as strong at night as at noon. Pitta digests dinner after you go to bed, but since the body is asleep, the heat is expended to keep you warm and to fuel the rebuilding of tissues, which occurs mostly at night. The Vata period in the early-morning hours expresses itself through the nervous system, but instead of thinking quickly as you do in the afternoon, you go into active dream sleep (called REM, or "rapid eye movement" sleep), when brain impulses are at their liveliest for the whole night. And thus the circle of the day is complete.

ONE DAY IN PERFECT RHYTHM

If you learn to ride these large waves of Vata, Pitta, and Kapha, your body will instinctively tune its subcycles, its many wheels within wheels, to follow suit. What would it be like to live a day in perfect rhythm? Ayurveda provides an ideal schedule called the *dinacharya*, or daily routine, that shows us how to find out.

DINACHARYA: THE DAILY ROUTINE

Four pivotal times set the rhythm of the entire daily cycle:

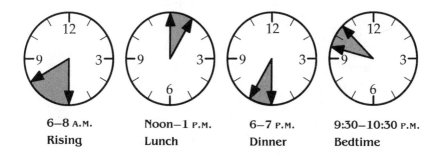

| 6–8 A.M. | Noon–1 P.M. | 6–7 P.M. | 9:30–10:30 P.M. |
| Rising | Lunch | Dinner | Bedtime |

The hours given are for starting an activity—the morning begins between 6 and 8 A.M., lunch begins anywhere from noon to 1 P.M., and so on. These times are approximate and change with the seasons. Ayurveda would prefer that you follow the sun and rise an hour before dawn every day of the year. By getting up during a Vata period, you take advantage of Vata's qualities of lightness, exhilaration, and freshness. These are infused into your body just before sunrise and last throughout the day.

Waiting too long into the Kapha period that follows (6 to 10 A.M.) causes you to wake up feeling duller, heavier, and less fresh. These qualities will also follow you all day; indeed, if you are a late riser year after year, you will train these Kapha qualities into your doshas and you will feel chronically "sleepy."

If you wanted to map out the ideal day, it would arrange itself naturally around the four pivotal points:

Rising: 6–8 A.M.

- Wake up without an alarm clock
- Drink a glass of warm water (to encourage regular morning bowel movements)
- Urinate; move your bowels (without forcing)
- Brush your teeth
- Clean your tongue if coated
- Massage your body with sesame oil (abhyanga)
- Bathe (in warm water, not too hot or cold)
- Exercise: Sun Salute (page 326)
- Yoga positions (page 339)
- Balanced breathing (Pranayama, page 360)
- Meditate
- Eat breakfast
- Take a mid-morning walk (for one-half hour)

Lunch: Noon–1 P.M.

- Eat lunch early (it should be largest meal of the day)
- Sit quietly for five minutes after eating
- Walk to aid your digestion (5 to 15 minutes)
- Meditate in the late afternoon

Dinner: 6–7 P.M.

- Eat a moderate dinner
- Sit quietly for five minutes after eating
- Walk to aid your digestion (5 to 15 minutes)

Bedtime: 9:30–10:30 P.M.

- Engage in light activity in the evening
- Get to bed early, but at least three hours after dinner
- Do not read, eat, or watch TV in bed

Naturally this is a very full schedule, but I hasten to say that hundreds of our patients (and their families) observe the dinacharya and have abundant time left over to pursue active lives. If you hesitate to modify your schedule, rest assured that you can be as busy as a doctor if you know how to ride nature's waves. The whole point of making the day orderly is that all your activity becomes healthier, more enjoyable, and more efficient. You gain more time than you lose, and it is quality time.

You will note that the main exercises are walking, plus gentle yoga poses coupled with meditation. Most of the other points are self-explanatory. I would just like to make a few additional points about each period of the day.

RISING: 6–8 a.m.

Morning is a special time in Ayurveda, when nature sends out its most delicate messages and you are most sensitive to them. Your nervous system has been built so that the sight of dawn, the still air on your skin, the faint sounds of birds and animals awakening, all set the stage for renewal. Alert to the slightest influence, the whole body is silent and poised in a delicate balance.

When you wake up, you should feel alert and clearheaded with no worries lingering from the day before, indicating that your nervous system is ready to be renewed. It is harmful to disturb or ignore this one opportunity to be naturally re-created. Writer Joan Mills has beautifully expressed the specialness of early rising: "From dawn's simplicities arise moments that are profound past explaining and powerful beyond sentiment. There are mornings when some small, isolated joy carries more conviction than a month of woe."

Medically speaking, the body precisely calibrates the correct biochemical balance for a full day's activities. It also empties the system of wastes from the previous day, which is why morning elimination is valuable before starting the new day's cycle. Having a bowel movement at this time is something you can gently encourage by drinking a glass of warm water and then allowing five minutes or so in the bathroom to see if your body wants to have a bowel movement. If not, don't worry about it. In time, if they keep this practice up regularly, most people find that an instinct for morning elimination will emerge.

When you brush your teeth, Ayurveda says that you should clean the white coating from the tongue if one has appeared overnight. This is the residue of ama, either from last night's meal or from a deeper imbalance. Not everyone wakes up with a coated tongue, so this step is optional. As your diet improves and you get into better balance, the coating tends to disappear.

The dinacharya asks you to do many different things in the early morning. It takes discipline to do all of them. You will be extending your routine by about an hour, which is a big change. But the rewards are big, too. When our patients stick to their morning routine in full, they report exhilarating health, unmatched by those who are careless or haphazard about it.

Try adding a few new elements to your present schedule and see how comfortable you feel with them. In order, the most important things to add are:

1. Early rising (at dawn)
2. Meditation
3. Ayurvedic exercises: Sun Salutes, Yoga positions
4. Oil massage

Meditation has already been discussed, and Ayurvedic exercises will be covered later, in a separate section. That leaves the oil massage (abhyanga), which is one of the most enjoyable parts of the dinacharya as well as a prime way to balance Vata dosha.

Lightly massaging the entire body with a thin film of oil before you bathe makes your skin feel warm and supple, a perfect balance for the cold dryness of Vata. Our Vata-type patients report that they are less prone to feel anxious or scattered during the day if they do their morning massage regularly. In fact, everyone would benefit enormously from balancing their Vata right at the start of the day. The skin contains thousands of cutaneous nerves that are connected to every part of the body. Science also recognizes that the skin is a major producer of endocrine hormones.

In scientific terms, your morning massage works by soothing the two master systems of the body, the nervous system and the endocrine system. No wonder that in ancient times Charaka lavished praise on the practice of abhyanga, holding that it rejuvenates the skin, tones the muscles, eliminates impurities, and promotes youthfulness. Massaging yourself is also a good way simply to start off the day relaxed, which Ayurveda considers extremely important. People who approach the day as a race against time do not have the best chance at perfect balance.

Here is how abhyanga is done.

HOW TO DO AN OIL MASSAGE (ABHYANGA)

Since this is a very light massage, it requires no more than a scant quarter cup of warm oil. Use a refined nut or seed oil sold in health-food stores. You can also order herbalized oils (page 378). Vata types do best with sesame or almond oil; Pittas respond to olive or coconut and Kaphas benefit from light or warm oils such as sunflower or sesame.

To heat the oil: Put three to four tablespoons of oil in a clear plastic cup or a squeeze bottle and set it in a bowl of very hot water. Wait a minute or two until the oil reaches skin temperature. Or, you can put the oil in a glass cup and heat it for ten to fifteen seconds in the microwave, *being very careful not to overheat it.*

Technically, it is best to use cured oil that has been subjected to high heat for only a brief period. You can carefully heat your oil to 212 degrees F, making sure that you watch it the whole time to prevent a possible fire.

The best place to perform your massage is in the bathroom. As good as it is for your body, there is no doubt that abhyanga is messy. No matter how careful you are, some oil will get splashed around. To minimize this, use a sheet of plastic (from a disposable trash bag) to cover the floor while you do your massage. Or put a small plastic stool in your tub and do your massage there. The mini-massage given at the end of this section is also less messy.

FULL BODY MASSAGE (5–10 MINUTES)

Start with your head: Pour a tablespoon of warm oil on your scalp. Using the flat of your hand and fingers, massage the oil in vigorously. Cover your entire scalp with small circular strokes, as if you were shampooing. Move to your face and ears, massaging more gently. Gentle massage of the temples and backs of the ears is especially good for settling Vata dosha.

Apply a little oil to your hands and massage your neck, front and back, then your shoulders. Use the flat of your palm and fingers.

Vigorously massage your arms, using a circular motion at the shoulders and elbows and long, back-and-forth motions on the long parts.

It is important not to be too vigorous when you get to your trunk. Using large, gentle circular motions, massage the chest, stomach, and lower abdomen. (Ayurveda traditionally advises moving in a clockwise direction.) A straight up-and-down motion is used over the breastbone.

Apply a bit of oil to your hands and reach around without straining to massage your back and spine—use up-and-down motions, or whatever you can do.

Vigorously massage your legs as you did your arms—circular at the ankles and knees, straight back-and-forth on the long parts.

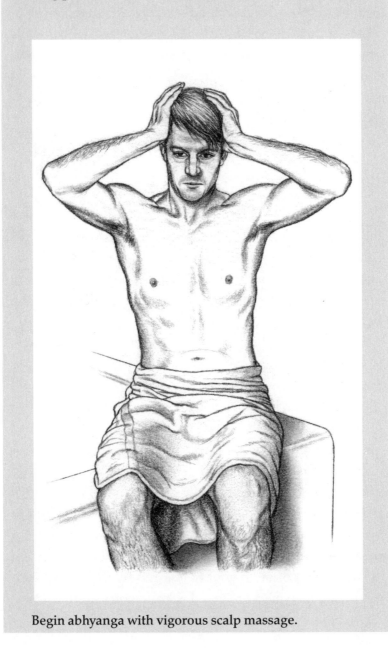

Begin abhyanga with vigorous scalp massage.

With the remaining bit of oil, vigorously massage your feet and toes.

Washing off the oil: Keeping a thin, almost undetectable film of oil on the body is considered very beneficial for toning the skin, balancing Vata, and keeping the muscles warm during the day. Therefore, you should wash yourself with warm, not hot, water and mild soap. If you look good with glossy hair, leave a bit of oil on your scalp, too, but most people will need to use shampoo.

MINI-MASSAGE (1–2 MINUTES)

Doing a full-body abhyanga sometimes takes too long for everyone's morning schedule, but it is so beneficial that we would rather have you do a short massage than none at all. The most important parts of the body to cover are the head and feet. They can be worked while you sit on the edge of the tub for a minute in the morning. This mini-massage takes only about two tablespoons of oil.

Take one tablespoon of warm oil and rub it into your scalp, using the same small, circular motions described above. Use the flat of your hand, and your fingertips.

Massage the forehead from side to side with your palm.

Gently massage your temples, using circular motions, then gently rub the outside of the ears.

Massage the back and front of your neck.

Taking the second tablespoon of oil, massage both feet using the flat of your hand. Work oil around your toes with your fingertips. Vigorously massage the soles of the feet with brisk back-and-forth motions of your palms. Sit quietly for a few seconds to relax and soak in the oil, then bathe normally.

LUNCH: NOON–1 P.M.

To catch the Pitta time of day at its height, it is best to eat lunch early, at noon or just before. Pitta stokes *agni*, the digestive fire, to its brightest at this hour; therefore, Ayurveda recommends that lunch be the biggest meal of the day. Since most people do not perform heavy physical labor, lunch does not have to be huge and hearty. Simply eat what you normally would for dinner.

To avoid becoming drowsy in the afternoon, do not drink alcohol at noon; warm water is the beverage that best promotes good digestion. In any event, minimize iced tea, ice water, or very cold soft drinks. All of these put out agni and make it harder to digest the meal.

Two other steps will remind the body of its daily rhythm. The first is to sit quietly for five minutes at the table after you finish eating, preferably in silence. The second is to take a short walk outside or to lie down for five minutes after the meal. Both stabilize the system and help start the process of digestion.

DINNER: 6–7 P.M.

Just after you come home from work is the time for afternoon meditation. You can prepare for it with a set of yoga positions and five minutes of balanced breathing, just as in the morning. Lying down for a few minutes beforehand also removes the jagged edge of a long workday and makes the meditation much deeper.

As with lunch, dinner comes early in order to catch a good time in the daily cycle. In this case, six o'clock is the beginning of a Kapha period, when the body wants to settle down. It is not a good idea to put too much fuel into your system at this time, since Pitta will not be along to digest your dinner until ten at night, when you are in bed. Your greatest digestive power is in the afternoon, which also allows ample time for complete digestion. Ayurveda is very strong on making sure that digestion is complete, since half-digested food is what creates ama.

Dinner should be a smaller meal than lunch. For many people, a bowl of hot soup with toast, herb tea, and fresh fruit are adequate. You are probably not used to eating lighter at dinner than lunch, but try it for a change. You'll be pleasantly surprised at how settled and comfortable your body feels when it doesn't have to digest full rations at night. Ayurveda cautions against fermented foods such as cheese, sour cream, and yogurt at night; red meat is best avoided since it is harder to digest.

Warm water or herb tea is the beverage of choice at dinner. Ayurveda makes no bones about considering alcohol a toxin that has no place in a healthy life, but I recognize that many people drink liquor after work. The basic rule is not to drink alcohol by itself, and don't have it ice cold. It is best to eliminate the cocktail hour altogether and eat an earlier dinner. Alcohol consumption with your meal should be light—a glass of wine, for example, or one beer.

A short walk after dinner helps promote digestion and prepares the system for a quiet evening spent reading, listening to music, or talking with friends and family. Avoid action-packed movies and TV late at night, since you don't want too much stimulation before bedtime.

BEDTIME: 9:30–10:30 P.M.

In order to get up at dawn, your bedtime has to be early. Attuned to the Kapha cycle that ends the evening, Kapha types already favor going to bed around ten; this is the Ayurvedic ideal for everyone. It allows the body's rhythms to slow down naturally, gives a deeper, more relaxing sleep, and provides time for the body to generate new tissue, which happens mostly at night. (I have already mentioned that getting a full night's sleep has been correlated with longevity.)

If you wait much past ten o'clock, the ensuing Pitta period will make you want to be active again—that is why people feel drowsy early in the evening, only to get a surge of energy around midnight, the absolute height of the Pitta period. Going to bed early is basically an all-or-nothing proposition, as far as your body rhythms are concerned. Therefore, I encourage you to try to get to bed at the Ayurvedic time. A week of self-discipline can be a revelation in terms of how good you feel the next day. To experience a day in perfect rhythm, you need a night of perfect sleep.

CHAPTER 12

DIET—EATING FOR PERFECT BALANCE

In Ayurveda, a balanced diet does not revolve around fats, carbohydrates, and proteins. Nor are calories, vitamins, and minerals given direct attention. We know these nutrients intellectually, not through direct experience. You cannot detect the vitamin C in your orange juice, much less the difference between it and vitamin A. For the most part, Western nutrition comes out of laboratory analysis. Ayurvedic nutrition comes directly from nature. When your taste buds greet a bite of food, an enormous amount of useful information is delivered to the doshas. Working solely with this information, Ayurveda allows us to eat a balanced diet naturally, guided by our own instincts, without turning nutrition into an intellectual headache.

When food talks to your doshas, it says many things, because the different gunas—heavy and light, dry and oily, hot and cold—are present in it. But the primary information is contained in its taste. Ayurveda recognizes six tastes, or rasas: sweet, sour, salty, and bitter are the four we already know, plus two others, pungent and astringent. All spicy food is pungent.

Astringent is the taste that puckers your mouth. The tannin in tea is astringent, as is the dry, mealy taste of beans.

In Ayurveda a balanced diet must contain all six rasas at every meal. The following dinner menu would be balanced:

Bibb lettuce salad (Bitter, Astringent)
Barbecued chicken with steamed rice (Salty, Sour, Pungent, Sweet)
Vanilla ice cream (Sweet)

Even if you eliminate the ice cream for dessert, this meal will remain in balance, since it still has all six tastes. If the barbecued chicken was replaced by baked chicken, the rasas of pungent and sour would be missing; they could be made up by adding a few slices of tomato (sweet and sour) and radish (pungent) to the salad.

It is not necessary to overload a meal with each taste. Just a hint of herbs and spices will add pungent and bitter to a meal. Nor is it good to let the same tastes dominate day after day. The basic rule is simply to give the body all six rasas at each meal so that it can respond to food completely.

SATISFYING THE DOSHAS

Taste can also be used to balance an aggravated dosha, since each dosha is on the lookout for the tastes that bring it into balance.

Vata is balanced by *salt*, sour, and sweet.
Pitta is balanced by *bitter*, sweet, and astringent.
Kapha is balanced by *pungent*, bitter, and astringent.

(The italicized taste has the strongest effect in decreasing a dosha.)

This basic information opens the door for a wealth of knowledge about what your body type should eat. In the following sections, we will expand upon this immense field. Our discussion covers the following subjects:

BODY-TYPE DIETS:

Vata	page 262
Pitta	page 270
Kapha	page 276
The Six Tastes	page 283
Agni—The Digestive Fire	page 293
A Blissful Diet	page 306

BODY-TYPE DIETS

The most basic guide to what you should eat is your body type. If you are a Vata, this dosha wants to be balanced with tastes different from those of either a Pitta or a Kapha. Let's say that two people are eating lunch at an outdoor cafe and both order a chef salad, iced tea, and lemon sherbet. If one person is a Pitta, this is an excellent lunch, for the sweet tastes and coolness of the food help balance Pitta dosha. But if the other person is a Vata, this meal is not good at all. Raw greens, particularly if bitter, cool drinks, and the lack of solid nourishment all throw Vata out of balance. When lunch is over, the two people will walk away feeling different, even though they ate the same meal. The Pitta will feel buoyant and refreshed, the Vata will feel unsatisfied and unenergetic.

That is why it is important to match your prakruti, your natural makeup, with the correct diet. Following is a table of food qualities as they affect the doshas.

BALANCES VATA		AGGRAVATES VATA	
Sweet	Heavy	Pungent	Light
Sour	Oily	Bitter	Dry
Salty	Hot	Astringent	Cold

BALANCES PITTA		AGGRAVATES PITTA	
Sweet	Cold	Pungent	Hot
Bitter	Heavy	Sour	Light
Astringent	Dry	Salty	Oily

BALANCES KAPHA		AGGRAVATES KAPHA	
Pungent	Light	Sweet	Heavy
Bitter	Dry	Sour	Oily
Astringent	Hot	Salty	Cold

As you can see, each section contains three tastes and three gunas, or qualities. The six tastes you already know: sweet, sour, salty, bitter, pungent, and astringent. The six gunas, which come in pairs, are:

- Heavy or light—wheat is heavy, barley is light, beef is heavy, chicken is light, cheese is heavy, skim milk is light
- Oily or dry—milk is oily, honey is dry, soybeans are oily, lentils are dry, coconut is oily, cabbage is dry
- Hot or cold (heats or cools the body)—pepper is hot, mint is cold, honey is hot, sugar is cold, eggs are hot, milk is cold

These qualities speak directly to the tongue and stomach. The operative principle is *"like speaks to like."* If you want to balance Pitta, avoid food that shares its qualities. A chili pepper, being pungent, hot, and oily, will naturally cause Pitta to become aggravated.

It is not necessary to memorize these qualities. Although Ayurvedic texts offer long lists of foods matched to their tastes and gunas, this knowledge is already built into your body. If you are in balance, you will want hot food when you feel cold, light food when you feel heavy. The same is true of taste. If you are a Kapha type, having a taste for green salads would tell you that you are in balance, because greens are generally bitter and astringent (these are two tastes that are good for you).

In a nutshell, that is what living in tune with nature means—what you like to eat is what your body needs for balance. On the other hand, if you are the same Kapha person and exclusively crave potato chips (salty), ice cream (sweet), and cheese (sour), your instincts are not in balance, and neither will be your Kapha dosha. The simple remedy is to start eating all six tastes again, moving away from your cravings. This will start to bring you back into balance, and as that happens, you will naturally regain your lost instincts. You won't abandon ice cream and potato chips, but a green salad will satisfy you just as much, because it satisfies your dominant dosha.

How to Choose the Right Body-Type Diet

Now that you know the general principles behind a balanced Ayurvedic diet, we can look at the specifics of each body type. Choosing which diet to follow is quite easy.

1. *Choose the diet that balances your dominant dosha.* If you are a pure Vata, for example, you will generally follow a Vata-pacifying diet. The same is true if you are a Vata-Pitta, although you can lean in the direction of the Pitta diet when you need to (during hot weather or if you display signs of Pitta aggravation, for instance).

If you are undecided about which of two doshas you should pacify, reflect on what foods you naturally favor that make you feel healthy and balanced. These will generally point you in the direction of the right diet. If you are one of the rare three-dosha types, you can usually eat any kind of Ayurvedic diet and remain in balance, but once again, let your instincts, the season of the year, and the state of your health be your guide.

2. If an Ayurvedically trained doctor has told you to balance a specific dosha, follow that diet.
3. Lean your diet in the direction indicated by the season of the year. Changes of season require certain modifications in your basic diet (you wouldn't drink iced tea in winter, for example, even if you are a strong Pitta type). These seasonal changes are covered in chapter 14, "Seasonal Routine."

Vata-Pacifying Diet

Favor:
Warm food, moderately heavy textures
Added butter and fat
Salt, sour, and sweet tastes
Soothing and satisfying foods

Vata is a cold, dry dosha, and the warm, nourishing foods we associate with winter—hearty stews and soups, slow-cooked casseroles, fresh-baked bread and fruit pies—give a good diet that soothes this dosha. At the opposite end of the spectrum, the foods we gravitate to in summer—cold salads, iced drinks, raw vegetables and greens—are not very congenial to it. Vata types tend to have erratic digestion, so soft, thoroughly cooked food that is easily digested helps them.

Vata dosha is also very sensitive to the atmosphere surrounding a meal. The best food in the world will not be good for you if tension at the table is curdling your stomach. Anything that makes dining a calmer, more restful experience will help to pacify Vata dosha.

❖

The Vata-pacifying diet given here is the first choice for all Vata types, unless diagnosis by a Ayurvedically trained physician has indicated something else. Within a few days of beginning this diet, you should definitely notice that your energy level is steady and that you feel more balanced, calmer, and happier. If you suffer from mild symptoms of Vata imbalance, such as insomnia, nervousness, or worry, this diet is also a natural choice. Try it for two weeks and see if your symptoms are alleviated.

We find that the following points are helpful when you start a Vata-pacifying diet.

- All soothing foods are generally good for settling disturbed Vata: milk (preferably warm), cream, butter, warm soups and long-cooked stews, hot cereals, and fresh-baked bread. All contain sweet, the most soothing taste to the body; most are also warm and heavy.
- A nourishing breakfast, the more substantial the better, will improve Vata throughout the day. Cream of rice or wheat is the best hot cereal for Vata, but anything warm, milky, and sweet is beneficial.
- Many Vata types experience a drastic energy slump in the late afternoon. Having hot tea with cookies or some other sweet is a good idea. Think of the four o'clock English teatime. Herb tea is more soothing than regular tea, whose high caffeine content can disturb Vata types. You

can try brewing gotu kola tea. This Indian herb, which is said to be excellent for calming the nerves, is available in health-food stores. You can also order Ayurvedic tea in bags (page 377). If you take five minutes for your tea break in a quiet spot before heading home from work, you will find the end of the day much less tiring.

- Pungent is not among the favored Vata tastes, but spicy food generally turns out to be satisfying to Vata types, because most spicy Mexican or Indian food is warm and has abundant oil in it. Ginger is the best pungent spice for Vata and is often used to improve Vata digestion (see page 301). Also, the use of sweet spices, such as cinnamon, fennel, and cardamom, helps restore a dull appetite, from which Vatas tend to suffer.

- Warm, moist food is very settling for Vata. Cooked grains and cereals are the best choices here. When you feel nervous, worried, or otherwise under pressure, a bowl of hot oatmeal or a cup of creamed vegetable soup will make you feel much better than a candy bar or a drink.

- Although sweet is good for Vata, sugar eaten by itself gives a quick energy boost that can make Vatas feel too restless. Warm milk is a sweet food in itself; it is very good for Vata, particularly with a little sugar or honey. Sugary sweets should be eaten in combination with nourishing ones like milk.

- Dry, salty snacks are not as good for Vata as salted nuts, which are heavier and oily, two qualities that pacify Vata. Almonds are the best choice. Ayurveda always recommends that almonds be skinned before they are eaten; standard advice is to soak a dozen whole almonds in water overnight, then peel and eat them in the morning to balance Vata. Since nuts and seeds are difficult to digest, Vatas need to eat them in small quantities, preferably ground into butters. Tahini (sesame paste) is an excellent source of sesame oil, one of the best foods for warming up and balancing Vata.

- All sweet fruits are good for Vata, and green grapes and mangoes are the best. Astringent fruits such as apples and pears need to be cooked before eating. Unripe fruit, being very astringent, is to be avoided, especially unripe bananas.

- Any cold, light, low-calorie food increases Vata and makes you feel dissatisfied. If you are partial to salads, let them come to room temperature and add oily dressing to make them more balancing. The same holds for raw vegetables. Eat them sparingly and not ice cold. In general, you should cook all your vegetables with a little oil rather than steaming them. This will make many "wrong" vegetables more acceptable to Vata dosha.

- When you go out for dinner, ask for warm water to sip in place of ice water, take the hot soup instead of salad, and feel free to eat bread and butter, as well as dessert (preferably a warm dessert like apple pie, rather than ice cream, whose coldness hampers Vata digestion).

- A hot breakfast cereal for dinner, although not the usual thing, tastes extremely good to anyone suffering from a Vata attack. Rice served with buttered lentils is also very good, as is a hearty minestrone-style soup. Pasta in all forms is very soothing. Warm milk before going to bed is a good idea, but eating very late at night is not—it may help you fall asleep, but your body will feel worse in the morning.

- Lassi, a traditional Indian drink, is good for ridding the body of excess Vata. To make it, whisk together one-half cup plain yogurt and one-half cup water; flavor with a pinch of powdered ginger, salt, or cumin. Sweet mango lassi, made from equal parts yogurt and mango pulp (fresh or canned) is particularly delicious and also balances Vata. For a lighter beverage, either lassi can be diluted with between one-half and one cup of water. One efficient and instant way to settle Vata is to sprinkle a special spice powder, called a Vata churna, over your plate at the table. An Internet source for churnas is on page 378.

Vata-Pacifying Foods

Vegetables

FAVOR	REDUCE
asparagus	broccoli
beets	Brussels sprouts
carrots	cabbage
cucumber	cauliflower
green beans	celery
okra	leafy green vegetables
onions and	mushrooms
garlic (not raw)	peas
radishes	peppers
sweet potatoes	potatoes
turnips	sprouts
	zucchini
	(These are acceptable if cooked with oil.)

Fruits

FAVOR	REDUCE
apricots	apples
avocados	cranberries
bananas	pears
berries	pomegranates
cherries	*(These are more acceptable if cooked.)*
coconut	Dried fruits in general; unripe fruit
dates	*(especially bananas)*
figs	
grapes	
mangoes	
melons	
nectarines	
oranges	
papayas	
peaches	
pineapple	
plums	
stewed fruits	
sweet, well-ripened fruit in general	

Grains

FAVOR	REDUCE
oats (cooked, not dry)	barley
rice	buckwheat
wheat	corn
	dry oats
	millet
	rye

Dairy

All dairy is acceptable, unless you have a known lactase deficiency.

Meat

FAVOR	REDUCE
chicken	red meat
seafood in general	
turkey	

Beans

FAVOR	REDUCE
chickpeas	All, except as noted.
mung beans	
pink lentils	
tofu	

Oils

All oils are acceptable; sesame oil is especially recommended.

Sweeteners

All sweeteners are acceptable.

Nuts and Seeds

All are acceptable in small amounts; almonds are best.

Herbs and Spices

FAVOR	REDUCE
Almost all, in moderation, with emphasis on sweet and/or heating herbs and spices, such as:	No spice should be used in large quantities; minimize all bitter and astringent herbs and spices, such as:

allspice	coriander
asafoetida	fenugreek
basil	parsley
bayleaf	saffron
black pepper	turmeric
caraway	
cardamom	
cilantro	
cinnamon	
clove	
cumin	
fennel	
ginger	
juniper berries	
licorice root	
marjoram	
nutmeg	
oregano	
sage	
tarragon	
thyme	

Pitta-Pacifying Diet

Favor:
Cool or warm but not steaming-hot foods
Moderately heavy textures
Bitter, sweet, and astringent tastes
Less butter and added fat

Pitta types are born with naturally strong, efficient digestion that remains that way unless disturbed. They come closest to the ideal of being able to eat a little of everything. Therefore, they need to be careful to avoid dietary abuses. The continued use of too much salt, overindulgence in sour and spicy food, and overeating are the most common aggravating influences.

Being the only hot dosha, Pitta appreciates cool foods, particularly in summer. It is a good idea to be especially scrupulous about having bitter and astringent tastes in your meals (supplied mainly through salads and legumes). These two rasas curb the appetite, dry up excessive moisture, and keep the palate sharp. They also counteract the dulling effect of too much salt and sugar on the taste buds, making it easier for Pittas to be moderate in their appetites, as nature intended them to be. Anything that makes dining a more soothing and orderly experience will also help to pacify this dosha.

The Pitta-pacifying diet given below is the natural choice for Pitta types, unless a Ayurvedically trained physician has indicated otherwise. Our Pitta patients report that they feel more balanced on this diet, still energetic but with a "softer" energy. Their roaring appetites calm down, too. If you suffer from mild symptoms of Pitta imbalance, such as heartburn, irritability, or excessive thirst, this diet is also good. Try it for a month and see if your symptoms are alleviated.

Some general points to help you implement this diet are as follows.

- Cool, refreshing food is best for Pitta types in summer, with a decrease in salt, oil, and spices, all of which are heating to the body. Salads contain two tastes, bitter and astringent, that balance Pitta and are also cold and light. Milk and ice cream are good, too.

- Excessive Pitta makes the body too sour; to counteract this, you should generally avoid pickles, yogurt, sour cream, and cheese. Fresh lemon juice is an exception and can be used, sparingly, instead of vinegar in your salad dressings. Fermented foods and alcoholic beverages are aggravating to Pitta because of their sourness, as are the acids in coffee. Learning to drink herb tea, either mint, licorice root, or the special Pitta-pacifying tea you can order (see page 378), will often make a big difference in smoothing your moods.

- A breakfast of cold cereal, cinnamon toast, and apple juice is a good replacement for coffee, doughnut, and orange juice, all of which disturb Pitta.

- The fat in red meat, which also heats the body, is not needed by Pitta people. Although they like to eat meat, particularly if they are high-powered movers and shakers, Pittas do better on a vegetarian diet than any other body type. If you are not vegetarian, make sure that your diet includes abundant amounts of milk, grains, and vegetables. All of these make Pittas feel extremely good. Once they become accustomed to health-food restaurants, Pittas like them better than their old steak houses because they feel calmer and more satisfied afterward.

- Fried foods are oily, hot, salty, and heavy, all qualities that Pittas need to avoid. On the other hand, starchy foods—vegetables, grains, and beans—are satisfying and cut ravenous Pitta hunger. The steady energy of a high-carbohydrate diet will counteract the tendency to overeat under stress.

- Processed and fast foods lean heavily on salt and sour tastes; it is a good idea for Pitta types to avoid them as much as possible. Since Pittas are fond of luxury, a subdued, elegant restaurant brings out the best in them. Japanese and Chinese food, being relatively low in fat and meat, are good choices for Pittas. When you eat out, order cool, not iced, water, take salad instead of hot soup, have the bread with a small amount of butter, and feel free to order dessert. Spicy food is too intoxicating to Pitta; if you like Mexican food, minimize the cheese and sour cream, and have a cool guacamole salad to counteract the heavy aggravation of Pitta caused by chilies.

- Pittas respond well to low-salt diets, but if forced to eat tasteless food, they will quickly rebel. Keeping salt off the table and adding it only in the kitchen while you cook is a good compromise. Cocktail hour with salty snacks is worse for Pitta types than anyone else. The dry, salty food and the alcohol combine to inflame their appetites and stomach linings.

- To bring down aggravated Pitta, a standard recommendation is to take two teaspoons of ghee (clarified butter) in a glass of warm milk. This also acts as a laxative, which helps flush excess Pitta from the system. Have your ghee and milk in place of dinner or two hours after a light dinner. You can also have it in place of breakfast. (Do not take ghee, however, if you have a problem with elevated cholesterol.)

- One efficient and instant way to settle Pitta is to sprinkle a special spice powder, called a Pitta churna, over your plate at the table. An Internet source for churnas is on page 378.

Pitta-Pacifying Foods

Vegetables

FAVOR

REDUCE

asparagus	garlic
broccoli	hot peppers
Brussels sprouts	onions
cabbage	radishes
cauliflower	tomatoes
celery	
leafy green vegetables	
lettuce	
mushrooms	
okra	
peas	
potatoes	
sprouts	
sweet peppers	
sweet potatoes	
zucchini	

Fruits

FAVOR

REDUCE

apples	apricots
avocados	berries
cherries	cherries (sour)
coconut	cranberries
figs	grapefruit
grapes	lemons
mangoes	persimmons
melons	
oranges	

Fruits (continued)

FAVOR	REDUCE
pears	Also avoid fruits that are sour or unripe.
plums	Grapes, oranges,
prunes	pineapples, and plums
raisins	should be sweet.

(All should be sweet and ripe.)

Grains

FAVOR	REDUCE
barley	brown rice
oats	corn
wheat	millet
white rice	rye

Dairy

FAVOR	REDUCE
butter	buttermilk
egg whites	cheese
ghee (clarified butter)	sour cream
ice cream	yogurt
milk	

Meats

FAVOR	REDUCE
chicken	Red meat and seafood in general.
shrimp	
turkey	

Beans

FAVOR	REDUCE
chickpeas	lentils
mung beans	
tofu and other soybean products	

Oils

FAVOR	REDUCE
coconut	almond
olive	corn
soy	safflower
sunflower	sesame

Sweeteners

All sweeteners are acceptable, except honey and molasses.

Nuts and Seeds

FAVOR	REDUCE
coconut	All, except as noted.
pumpkin seeds	
sunflower seeds	

Herbs and Spices

FAVOR

Spices are generally
reduced as heating, but
some sweet, bitter and
astringent ones are good
in small amounts, including:

cardamom
cilantro
cinnamon
coriander
dill
fennel
mint
saffron
turmeric

REDUCE

All pungent herbs and
spices, except as noted;
also take only small
amounts of:

barbecue sauce
catsup
sour salad dressing
mustard

Plus small amounts of cumin and black pepper

Kapha-Pacifying Diet

Favor:
Warm, light food
Dry food, cooked without much water
Minimum of butter, oil, and sugar
Pungent, bitter, and astringent tastes
Stimulating foods

Kapha is a slow dosha to be affected by food, but over time, Kapha types become imbalanced as a result of eating too many sweet, rich foods. Other problems can develop, but in Western society, where sugar and fat account for more than half of the calories consumed by the average person, Kaphas have to be on guard against this influence. Salt also needs to be watched, since it too is greatly overused and promotes fluid retention in many Kaphas.

Anything that increases lightness should be favored—a small, light meal at breakfast and dinner, lightly cooked foods (no deep-frying), raw fruits and vegetables. Eating spicy food will promote better digestion and warm your body; bitter and astringent foods will help to curb your appetite. In general, anything that makes eating stimulating will help balance Kapha and avert the danger, ever-present with most Kapha types, of overindulging at the table.

The Kapha-pacifying diet given below is the natural choice for Kapha body types, unless contrary advice has been given by a Ayurvedically trained physician. Switching to this diet helps many of our Kapha patients feel more balanced, energetic, lighter, and happier about themselves. If you suffer from mild symptoms of Kapha imbalance, such as a stuffed or runny nose, being slow to start in the morning, or oversleeping, this diet is also good. Try it for six weeks and see if your symptoms are alleviated.

The following suggestions will help people implement a Kapha-pacifying diet.

- Given a choice, pick hot food over cold at every meal—a hot luncheon entree instead of a sandwich, hot apple pie instead of ice cream, grilled fish instead of tuna salad. Warming up cold Kapha digestion is always good for balance. Dry cooking methods (baking, broiling, grilling, sautéing) are better for Kaphas than moist ones (steaming, boiling, poaching).

- Before you eat, stimulate your appetite with bitter or pungent tastes instead of salty or sour. The bitterness of romaine lettuce, endive, or tonic water will wake up your taste buds without encouraging you to overeat. Ginger tea or even a pinch of fresh gingerroot is also highly recommended. In general, you want to be sure that bitter and astringent tastes are present in every meal. To get them, it is not necessary to seek out bitter food in quantity. A little bitterness in a salad or the astringency of herbs supplies enough. Among the household spices, cumin, fenugreek, sesame seed, and turmeric are both bitter and astringent.

- Adding pungent tastes to your diet with spices is one of the best ways to balance Kapha. Anything spicy is good, including very hot Mexican or Indian food that makes your eyes water. This action flushes out all the mucous membranes. Contrary to what we tend to think, hot, spicy food is best not in the summer but in the winter; it offsets the cold, damp quality that Kapha resents.

- Kaphas need to eat breakfast mainly to get them started in the morning, not for solid nourishment. Rather than relying on a jolt of caffeine from coffee, wake your body up with light, Kapha-reducing foods, such as hot spiced cider, buckwheat pancakes with apple butter, corn muffins, and bitter cocoa made with skim milk and a touch of honey. In general, anything hot and light is good, while anything cold, heavy, or sweet is not so good. Cold cereals, cold juice or milk, and sugary pastries tend to create congestion, particularly in damp winter weather. Bacon and sausage are Kapha-aggravating because of their salt and oil. If you don't feel hungry in the morning, it is all right to skip breakfast, which Ayurveda considers optional, especially for Kapha types.

- If you wake up feeling congested in the morning, a sign of excess Kapha, the best things to take are honey, hot water, lemon juice, and ginger. Hot ginger tea (page 301) is excellent for Kapha types in general, since it stimulates the system and flushes out excess Kapha. If you occasionally skip a meal—a good idea for many Kaphas—a spoonful of honey in hot water will tide you over.

- Cutting back on sweets is difficult for many Kaphas, but a trial week on a low-sugar diet generally does result in feeling lighter and more energetic. Honey is extensively recommended for Kapha types, but you should not take more than a tablespoon or so per day; honey is not suitable to cook with, either, since heating honey makes it unwholesome, according to Ayurveda.

- Out-of-balance Kapha types overindulge in dairy products, but butter, ice cream, and cheese are among the worst for you, since they make your system colder and more congested. Low-fat milk is best, preferably pre-boiled to aid digestion, with only a minimum of other dairy products. Sesame seeds on rolls and bread help to counteract the sweet, heavy quality of the wheat, which is not the best for Kapha, either. Because they combine too much heavy sweetness, a hamburger and milkshake, or even a sandwich with milk, should be eaten only infrequently.

- Raw fruits, vegetables, and salads are extremely good, since their fiber tones the intestinal tract, in addition to the benefits of their astringent tastes. Generally speaking, Ayurveda prefers all food cooked, but we find that this is an exception that helps most Kapha types.

- Deep-fried foods of any kind will aggravate Kapha; they are among the few things you should try to eliminate from your diet. There is no need to banish all fats, but make an effort to use less butter and oil in your cooking. Corn oil is heating to the body; it is a good choice for you in small quantities, along with almond and sunflower oils. Crisp-steamed vegetables with a little ghee (clarified butter) drizzled over them is good for a light supper; anything crisp, fresh, and stimulating balances Kapha.

- Restaurant food has to be carefully chosen by Kapha people. Fast food is far too oily, salty, and sweet—head for the salad bar and use a minimum of salad dressing. If you are eating out in better restaurants, Oriental cooking is the lightest, particularly if you concentrate on more vegetables than meat. Wherever you go, order a glass of hot water instead of iced, take salad instead of hot soup (except in cold weather), avoid the rolls and butter, and make dessert small and not too rich—hot fruit pies are probably the best choice.
- One efficient and instant way to settle Kapha is to sprinkle a special spice powder, called a Kapha churna, over your plate at the table. An Internet source for churnas is on page 378.

Kapha-Pacifying Foods

Vegetables

FAVOR	REDUCE
Generally all, including:	Sweet and juicy vegetables, such as:
asparagus	
beets	sweet potatoes
broccoli	tomatoes
Brussels sprouts	zucchini
cabbage	
carrots	
cauliflower	

FAVOR

celery
eggplant
garlic
leafy green vegetables
lettuce
mushrooms
okra
onions
peas
peppers
potatoes
radishes
spinach
sprouts

Fruits

FAVOR	REDUCE
apples	avocados
apricots	bananas
cranberries	coconuts
pears	dates
pomegranates	fresh figs
	mangoes
Dried fruits in general	melons
(apricots, figs, prunes, raisins).	oranges
	papayas
	peaches
	pineapples
	Sweet, sour, or very juicy
	fruits in general.

Grains

FAVOR	REDUCE
barley	oats
buckwheat	rice
corn	wheat
millet	
rye	

Dairy

FAVOR	REDUCE
Low and non-fat milk and dairy in small amounts	All, except as noted.

Meat

FAVOR	REDUCE
chicken	Red meat and seafood in general.
shrimp	
turkey	

Beans

FAVOR	REDUCE
All legumes are acceptable.	Reduce kidney beans and tofu.

Oils

FAVOR	REDUCE
almond	All, except as noted.
corn	
safflower	
sunflower	

Sweeteners

FAVOR	REDUCE
Raw, unheated honey.	All, except as noted.

Nuts and Seeds

FAVOR	REDUCE
pumpkin seeds	All, except as noted.
sunflower seeds	

Herbs and Spices

FAVOR	REDUCE
All—ginger is best for improving digestion.	salt

THE SIX TASTES

Each of the six tastes speaks directly to the quantum mechanical body, and each carries a different message. Our tongues know this instinctively. The voluptuous sweetness of vanilla custard is diametrically opposed to the bitter bite of lemon peel; one is soothing, the other is a shock. Your whole body reacts to the difference, which begins on your tongue but continues throughout your body. Taste leaves a trail of reactions from your mouth to the food's final destination, your cells.

Without knowing about nutritional balance in terms of fats, carbohydrates, and proteins, native cultures around the world have realized that their diets had to be dynamic. They had to have tastes that wake up the body, like bitter and astringent, and others that soothe it, primarily sweet. Digestion sometimes needed to be increased with "hot" tastes—pungent, sour, and salty—and at other times decreased with "cold" tastes—bitter, astringent, and sweet.

All of this was understood instinctively. In Mexico, the limited fare of corn and beans could not by itself have supported a healthy, balanced existence, but with the addition of red chilies, it has served the native people for many centuries. Red chili adds vitamin C to a diet, but the more important addition it brings are the sweet and pungent tastes that round out the six rasas. Curry spices serve the same purpose in India, where the staples of rice, lentils, and wheat bread would be dramatically limited without them.

MESSAGES FROM NATURE

Every food has its own profile of tastes. Simple foods, such as white sugar or vinegar, have only one taste, but most others have at least two: lemon is sour, but also sweet and bitter; carrots are sweet, bitter, and astringent; cheese is sweet and sour. Milk is considered a complete food, having the subtle presence of all six rasas besides its obvious sweetness; for this reason, Ayurveda recommends drinking milk alone rather than combining it with a meal. (Having milk with other sweet foods—fruit, grains, and sugar—is good, however; in fact, milk is the best buffer for refined white sugar, which enters the system in a rush if digested alone.)

The major food groups all revolve around the rasa of sweet, but with the five other tastes carefully blended in:

Fruits—primarily sweet and astringent, with citrus fruits adding sour

Vegetables—primarily sweet and astringent, with leafy greens adding bitter

Dairy—primarily sweet, with yogurt and cheese adding sour and astringent

Meat—primarily sweet and astringent

Oils—primarily sweet

Grains and Nuts—primarily sweet

Legumes—primarily sweet and astringent

Herbs and Spices—primarily pungent, with all other flavors added secondarily

Just as most foods are sweet, so is Kapha dosha, the builder of tissues; the human body as a whole is therefore sweet, too. Herbs and spices fill in the spectrum of tastes, but, more important, they evoke a complete range of bodily responses. Black pepper makes your mouth water, fenugreek dries it up; mustard heats the body, mint cools it off. The only blank space is salt, which is provided by salt itself.

Using its taste profile, every food can be described as either increasing or decreasing one or more doshas, as we saw. Since the three doshas are connected, an increase of one is so crucial that Ayurveda has described every food according to whether it will increase or decrease a particular dosha. Cabbage, for instance, is known to increase Vata, onions to increase Pitta, all oils to increase Kapha.

Considering that half a dozen messages are being relayed to the body simultaneously by any one food, you can get just as strong a headache computing the six rasas as trying to compute every gram of fat, carbohydrate, and protein. This complex job belongs to a Ayurvedic doctor. To him, food is medicine, and its properties must be scrutinized as closely as any other medicine. He needs to know that cabbage is sweet and astringent, dry and cooling, and therefore a strong aggravator of Vata (that is why cabbage tends to form gas in the colon, the seat of Vata). He would then be able to prescribe an offsetting food (such as fennel) to counteract Vata aggravation.

He also knows that every food delivers an "aftertaste" (*vipak*) that affects the body once the food has been digested. Cabbage's aftertaste is pungent, for example. Vipak is an important consideration when a doctor is prescribing a therapeutic diet, because he needs to know every aspect of the food that is affecting his patient's doshas. At home you do not have to be so specific. The aftertaste of food once it has been digested is something we will leave to the doctor, but for the sake of completion, vipak is classified as follows:

Sweet and salty tastes lead to sweet vipak
Sour taste leads to sour vipak
Pungent, bitter, and astringent tastes lead to pungent vipak

Thus the six tastes are reduced to three after digestion is completed.

In the following pages we delve more deeply into the six rasas and what they say to your doshas. I hope you will read this section at least once, but do not memorize it. Your taste buds, not your mind, should be the final judge of taste.

Sweet

Sweet foods:

Sugar, honey	Increases Kapha (except honey)
Rice	Decreases Pitta and Vata
Milk, cream, butter	
Wheat bread	

Sweet is a taste that strongly increases Kapha. Eating sweet foods will bring on Kapha qualities in the body—coldness, heaviness (by adding fat), steadiness, and physical energy. Just as Kapha people are naturally the most easily satisfied, sweet is the most satisfying taste. It is very Kapha to be sweet-natured and motherly—from childhood on, two Kapha foods, milk and sugar, represent motherliness. Any food that feels nourishing and brings satisfaction generally has a sweet component. For instance, all meats, oils, and most grains are considered sweet. Ayurveda looks upon rice and wheat, the two grains that are the staff of life in the East and West, as sweet in taste. Ghee (clarified butter) is another sweet food, being derived from milk; it is considered the best remedy for balancing Pitta.

Sweet foods are also soothing and relieve thirst. If you are in a nervous, unsettled mood, which is a sign of aroused Vata, sweet will calm you; it also puts out the fire of Pitta (an angry baby is pacified by giving it milk or sugar). However, too much sugar is not stabilizing; it makes the mind dull and drowsy. Complacency, greed, and emotional dependency come from too much sweet.

Too much sweet becomes cloying. It leads to negative qualities that come from pushing Kapha too far: sluggishness, overweight, mental dullness, excess mucus, congestion, and sleepiness. Kapha people are endowed with qualities of satisfaction and well-being that Vata and Pitta types have to seek through sweet tastes. However, in the case of any Kapha imbalance, sweet foods are considered undesirable and should be reduced or avoided. Only honey is an exception to this rule. It is better than any other sweet food for balancing Kapha.

Salt

Salty foods:

Salt   Increases Kapha and Pitta

                           Decreases Vata

Salt increases both Pitta and Kapha. It sparks digestion, a Pitta function. Its taste adds savor to food, stokes the appetite, and starts the flow of saliva and stomach juices. Salt is hot like Pitta (all the digestive processes heat up the body). Too much of it, however, and the other tastes are overwhelmed, making nothing taste good. The Kapha connection is through two other qualities Ayurveda associates with salt—oiliness and heaviness. By attaching itself to water molecules, salt makes your tissues heavier. Excessive salt will make it harder to control food cravings, which Kapha types must do to remain on a balanced diet. By making you eat too much, salt adds fat and leads to overweight.

In the West, the connection between salt and hypertension has been convincing enough that many patients with high blood pressure have been forbidden to eat any but the smallest amounts of salt. This implied that salt was somehow an enemy. Now it is known that such restrictions were too severe—a normal person can eat moderate amounts of salt without harm to his blood pressure. The basic reason not to overindulge is that a moderate diet promotes health in every way, not just by averting hypertension. Ayurveda would point out that salt doesn't raise blood pressure, the doshas do. It takes a dosha imbalance before the salt will do any harm.

Too much salt also leads to Pitta-related skin inflammation, acne, and overheating. If there is a Pitta or Kapha imbalance in the body, salty food is considered undesirable.

Emotionally, salt gives life its zest, but too much salt nullifies this effect, just as too many potato chips kills the appetite instead of stimulates it. If you overuse salt, it takes more and more of it to register at all—this is why salty foods are compulsive. Excess salt in general is associated with cravings and compulsive desires.

Sour

Sour foods:

Lemons	Increases Pitta and Kapha
Cheese, yogurt	Decreases Vata
Tomatoes, grapes,	
plums, other sour fruits	
Vinegar	

Like salt, sour is a Pitta-Kapha taste that sparks the digestion and adds savor to food. It is refreshing to eat sour food, but it increases thirst, which is connected to Pitta—the heat generated by extra Pitta has to be slaked with lots of water. Sour food can therefore add to fluid retention, making the body heavier (more Kapha). Pitta's sharp qualities, such as sharp intellect and wittiness, are increased by sour foods, but "turning sour" is also possible, since too much Pitta is connected with resentment and envy, popularly called "sour grapes."

Cheese and yogurt derive their sourness from fermentation. In small quantities, sour foods make the digestive juices flow.

However, Ayurveda is distinctly opposed to fermented sourness in general—vinegar and fermented alcohol are considered toxic, reflecting the Pitta-Kapha quality of this taste. Out-of-balance Pitta brings toxicity to the blood; out-of-balance Kapha makes the tissues stagnant with ama.

Excess of sour foods leads to acidic difficulties in the body, such as ulcers, disturbed blood chemistry, skin irritations, and heartburn. If there is a Pitta or Kapha imbalance in the body already, sour foods are considered undesirable. Fermented foods are undesirable at any time except in small amounts.

Bitter

Bitter foods:

Bitter greens (endive, chicory, romaine lettuce)	Increases Vata Decreases Pitta and Kapha
Bitter cucumbers	
Tonic water	
Lemon rind	
Spinach, leafy greens in general	
Turmeric, fenugreek	

Bitter is the most Vata of tastes, being light, cold, and dry in its effects on the body. It is a corrective taste, bringing the cravings for sweet, sour, and spicy foods back into balance. Bitter quickens the palate by waking it up, not by satisfying it, a very Vata property, since Vata is responsible for alertness. A dash of bitters or a glass of tonic water is effective in getting the digestion going for people with slow digestion; the bitterness instantly makes the palate want the more satisfying tastes.

Bitter tones the tissues, a property that gave tonic water its name. Bitter is the best taste, along with sweet, for cooling you off in hot weather. When the body has become toxic, inflamed, hot, or itchy as a result of Pitta aggravation, bitter is considered the best corrective. (Bitter quinine bark soothes fever, for example.)

In excess, bitter aggravates Vata, leading to typical Vata complaints—loss of appetite, weight loss, headaches, unsteadiness, dry skin, and a hollow feeling of weakness. The bracing alertness associated with bitter turns to bitter feelings in excess, associated with lack of satisfaction—anything that is too Vata is not satisfying, because Vata's nature is constantly to seek change. Grief, which destroys the balance of Vata and makes life seem completely without satisfaction, is bitter.

Pungent

Pungent foods:
Cayenne, chili peppers   Increases Vata and Pitta
Onions and garlic   Decreases Kapha
Radishes
Ginger
Spicy food in general

In Ayurveda, hot, spicy food is considered to have its own taste, called pungent. Pungency is immediately recognizable because it causes a burning sensation (the increased Pitta) and thirst (the drying effect of increased Vata). Pungency heats up the body and makes fluids flow out of it. As a result, digestion is increased and congested tissues are cleaned out. Sweat, tears, saliva, mucus, and the blood all start flowing when pungency is present.

Because it flushes out your sinus cavities, pungent food is the best for balancing Kapha, which when aggravated leads to congestion of mucous membranes. Western medicine long thought that spicy food must be bad for anyone with irritated mucous membranes, but the effect of opening and flushing out the tissues is now considered extremely beneficial; sufferers of chronic bronchitis and asthma have sometimes been put on Mexican food laden with chili pepper. The antitoxic effect of pungent is said to help clear the skin, even though Pitta is increased—the Vata dryness cleans out the oily pores that exacerbate acne.

In excess, pungency turns to pain—eating a raw chili causes swollen lips and eyes, burning skin, and hot sweat. Too much spicy food makes you overly thirsty, dizzy, and unsettled, reflecting the Vata influence (too much Vata makes for light-headedness and dryness). The sharpness of pungent, if pushed too far, will not excite the body but irritate it.

The same is true of the emotions. Pungent humor is invigorating, but it can also be sharp and hurtful. Excitable, extroverted people are already inclined to be pungent—if you add more, they turn feverish. If a Vata or Pitta imbalance is present in the body, pungent food is not desirable.

Astringent

Astringent foods:

Beans	Increases Vata
Lentils	Decreases Pitta and Kapha
Apples, pears	
Cabbage, broccoli, cauliflower	
Potatoes	

Astringent, the taste that makes your mouth dry and puckered, is the least familiar of the six rasas. It is an alkaline taste, equal but opposite to the puckering of sour lemons. Like bitter, astringent is Vata—the gas produced by boiled cabbage and the dry, mealy taste of beans are both Vata effects. Astringency is light like bitter but more appetizing; traditional cultures around the world have subsisted on beans, and in the Middle Ages, cabbage was a staple food throughout Europe. Astringency is settling; potatoes, carrots, and other earthy foods bring out this satisfying effect.

Astringent is cooling and constrictive; it stops the flow of secretions such as sweat and tears (making beans a good pairing for chili peppers, since they offset each other). In excess, its constricting effect may lead to Vata complaints of constipation and dry mouth, along with gas or distension in the lower abdomen.

People who have a dry wit are astringent. It is a quality that dampens excitement and brings you back to yourself. Taken too far, however, astringency becomes shriveling. The sudden constriction when you are seized by fear and the dry mouth that anxiety brings are both negative astringent qualities. Astringent emotions lack warmth in general; to be old, cold, and shriveled up is what makes people into old prunes if they age badly. If there is a Vata imbalance in the body, astringent food is undesirable.

AGNI—THE DIGESTIVE FIRE

Most people have never consulted a physician about their digestion. As a society used to good health, we take for granted our ability to process food, and, in the absence of a serious problem like peptic ulcers or colitis, we ignore the occasional upset stomach or uncomfortable night spent after "eating the whole thing."

Ayurveda, on the other hand, considers poor digestion a major factor in the disease process and extols good digestion as the giver of health. Every cell has been created from food. If the food has been used well, then the cells will be built well; if it has been used badly, then the disease process has already started. The Ayurvedic sages liked to say that if you could digest it properly, poison would be good for you, while with poor digestion, a person can die from drinking nectar.

DIGESTION AND THE DOSHAS

Ayurveda says that there are no absolutely good or bad foods, only food that is good or bad for *you*. Being able to extract every life-giving value from what you eat is of the utmost importance. People are not born equal in this regard— the three major body types have very different powers of digestion.

Vata digestion tends to be variable and often delicate.
Pitta digestion tends to be strong and intense.
Kapha digestion tends to be slow and often heavy.

As with everything that the doshas touch, each style of digestion has its advantages and drawbacks. Vatas may not be thrilled to discover that they tend to have delicate or unreliable digestion, but this makes them more discriminating eaters, and they rarely have to worry about the runaway appetites of Pittas or the discouraging slide into overweight experienced by many Kaphas. The important thing is to make maximum use of the digestion you were born with and improve it as much as possible.

The digestive tract not only extracts nutrition for your body, it is highly responsive to your emotions. Your "gut feelings" have been put there by nature so that the mind and body can communicate. Vata imbalance often shows up as disturbed feelings that create pain in the intestines. Pitta dosha is responsible for correct metabolism and "pure blood" (absence of tox-

ins); it is also the dosha that controls the proper rate of digestion. This is called *agni*, or "the digestive fire."

Agni is one of the most important principles in Ayurveda,
equal to the doshas. A primary sign of good health is that your
agni is burning bright, that is, you are digesting your food efficiently, distributing all the necessary nutrients to every cell,
and burning off waste products without leaving deposits of
toxins. Therefore, by balancing agni, one keeps all these things
in balance at the same time.

Nature has set up everyone's body in such a way that agni
follows a cycle throughout the day; unless agni's daily rhythm
is correctly set, digestion will suffer. One of the most valuable
things to know is how to reset a flickering agni and coax it
back into its natural groove.

How to Reset Agni

Agni's daily rhythm rises and falls, making you slightly
hungry in the morning, very hungry at noon, and moderately
hungry in the early evening. In between these times, agni
shuts down your appetite so that it can proceed to digest the
food you have already eaten. When your stomach is empty
again, agni renews your appetite once more.

If this basic cycle is thrown off, the body becomes confused—appetite and digestion start to overlap. Your agni will
tell you if this has happened by a wide range of symptoms:

- Heartburn and acid stomach
- Fluttering stomach or nervous digestion
- Loss of appetite at mealtimes
- Constipation or diarrhea
- Lack of interest in food
- Overweight or underweight

- Serious digestive disorders: irritable bowel syndrome, ulcers, diverticulitis, et cetera

The first and most important thing to do if any of these symptoms appears is to reset your agni to its natural cycle. It is also a good idea to do this just to tone your digestion, even if you have no digestive problems.

Vata types can reset agni once a month.

Pitta types can reset agni twice a month (it is also good to do it whenever your appetite has become ravenous and you begin to overeat).

Kapha types can reset agni up to once a week, unless there are serious digestive complaints. Kapha dosha benefits from this routine more than the other doshas, since digestion tends to be heavy and slow.

No matter what your body type, do not attempt to reset your agni if you are feeling sick. Being sick usually indicates that agni is down (or at least not running correctly); that is not a good time to be tampering with it. *If you have an ulcer, colitis, or any other serious digestive complaint*, do not restart agni, except under a doctor's care.

The method for resetting agni is as follows:

Weekend Program

It takes roughly two days to reset agni. Since rest is one of the requirements on the day you do not eat, doing the program over the weekend is best for most people.

FRIDAY ROUTINE

Eat normally at breakfast and lunch. Do not have an afternoon snack or any alcohol after noon. Eat a light dinner of nourishing food, making sure that it is satisfying but not heavy; exclude spicy food and cheese. Just before bedtime, take a laxative—three tablets of senna (Sennokot®), followed by a small glass of hot water. Go to bed early. Some people will wake up during the night for a bowel movement, others will wait until morning—either way is normal.

SATURDAY ROUTINE

Before you can reset your agni, it is necessary first to lower it. This is done by not eating meals and only drinking liquids during the day. Vata and Pitta types should drink fruit juice diluted with warm water. Apple or grape juice are good; orange juice is too acidic. Drink one glass of juice at breakfast, at lunch, and at dinnertime; three or four more can be taken between meals, but do not drink more than that unless it's water. The aim is to have no appetite and only a minimum of calories to digest. Kapha types can follow this routine *or* drink only warm water, if they are comfortable with that.

Spend the day reading, watching TV, or performing light activity. A short walk in the morning and in the afternoon is a good idea. Do not travel any distance or undertake heavy physical tasks. If you run or exercise heavily, skip it for a day and relax.

If you feel faint with hunger, take one tablespoon of honey with a glass of warm water and lie down for five minutes.

It is normal to feel lightness in your limbs, but if you start to tremble or feel dizzy, lie down and rest. If the feeling persists, eat a small meal. You may be unsettled from unusually high stress that has thrown you off balance.

SUNDAY ROUTINE

Now you want to restart your agni and let it adjust itself to its normal cycle. To do this, eat a light breakfast of hot cereal (oatmeal, cream of rice, or cream of wheat) with a little butter, milk, and sugar. Herb tea is also good in the morning to soothe the stomach—licorice root for Vatas, peppermint for Pittas and Kaphas. If you followed the program correctly on Saturday, this will be all the breakfast you'll want. If you still feel very hungry, have more cereal or a glass of juice. Coffee, tea, and cigarettes will throw off your agni rhythm and defeat your purpose. (Kapha types, who are slow starters in the morning, can drink gotu kola tea as a stimulant—this herb is sold in health-food stores.)

Do not eat again until noon.

At exactly noon, have a good lunch, one that satisfies you without being heavy or immoderate. It is best not to excite your digestion with salty or spicy food or alcohol, but do not have just a salad and water, either. Ginger tea is a good idea. If you are Vata and have no appetite, drink it before the meal; otherwise, during or after the meal is fine. If you do not have ginger tea, sip a glass of warm water with your meal.

Do not eat again until dinner.

Have an early dinner (at least three hours before you go to bed), eating a nourishing meal that suits your body type. Make this meal smaller than lunch. Rice, lentils, and steamed vegetables are good. Even a repeat of breakfast would be good for most Kaphas and Pittas, or for anyone who tends to overeat.

Now that your agni is reset, your hunger cycle will naturally tend to make you want

- a light breakfast
- a substantial lunch, *eaten at the same time every day*
- a light supper, *eaten early and at the same time every day*

The following things will throw your agni off again and should be avoided.

- *Eating between meals.* The rule here is not to stimulate your appetite if you are not going to eat. Agni likes to finish what it starts; therefore, it is thrown off by empty stimulation from chewing gum, hard candy, or breath mints taken throughout the day. However, having tea and cookies in the afternoon is a good idea for Vata types or for anyone who gets fatigued at the end of the workday.
- *Strong stimulants.* Caffeine, salt, and alcohol are strong stimulants and should be taken moderately. The indigestion most people feel at a cocktail party comes from the mixing of salty food, alcohol, and noise. If you like to drink coffee, always have it with food, not alone. The same applies to salt and alcohol. Being addicted to any of these stimulants makes it impossible to balance the digestion.
- *Skipping meals.* Agni wants something to do three times a day and resents it if you do not eat. Kapha types can skip meals because their agni moves slowly and burns low, but it is still a good rule to eat three times a day.

AGNI AND AMA

The Ayurvedic ideal is that agni be kept operating efficiently under all conditions; it must not be so cold that food is not completely digested. Partially digested food turns into ama, a cold, foul-smelling residue whose "stickiness" prevents the doshas from circulating freely as they should. There is also the opposite danger that agni will burn too high, in which case the nutrients in food will not be extracted but burned away. Then digestion becomes feverish, leading to weakness instead of strength.

Agni and ama form the most important pair of opposites in the body, making the difference between a state of dynamic health and a state of slow deterioration. The most obvious difference between the two is that agni makes you feel well, while ama makes you feel sick. There are some specific signs as well. Agni gives one:

- Glowing complexion and bright eyes
- Strong digestion without constipation or diarrhea
- Ability to eat all foods
- Clear, straw-colored urine
- Normal feces without strong smell

If there is ama in the body, it can vary from a minor to a major serious condition. Among the earlier signs are:

- Dull skin and eyes
- Unpleasant taste in the mouth, with coated tongue in the morning
- Strong bad breath
- Urine that is cloudy, dark, or discolored
- Weak digestion, chronic constipation and/or diarrhea
- Loss of appetite (food tastes bad)
- Aching joints

Once the digestive fire has returned to normal and the collected ama from the past is flushed out, agni by itself will continue to purify the body. Your digestion is self-correcting, because nature has set things up so that agni burns ama. This is another example of how you can trust your body to know what to do.

Certain foods, spices, and herbs are effective in improving the quality of agni in everyone, according to Ayurveda. They are used to stimulate appetite, increase the power of digestion, and remove ama.

GINGER

Dried into a powder or used fresh, ginger is praised as the best spice for helping the agni of all body types. Powdered ginger, sold in grocery-store spice racks, is stronger, more drying, and more pungent than fresh gingerroot, which is sold in the fresh produce department (or in health-food stores if your supermarket does not carry it). Fresh ginger is considered the better digestive aid.

Ginger can be used in various ways:

As a tea. Boil a large pinch of dry ginger in a cup of water over a low flame until a quarter of the water boils away, then strain. This tea is drunk before meals to whet the appetite. A small glass of it can be sipped during or after meals to aid digestion.

Fresh ginger tea is made by first boiling your water and then, with the heat off, dropping in a few thin slices of unpeeled gingerroot (about one tablespoon per cup of water). Allow to steep for five minutes, then strain. You can make a much stronger tea by boiling the slices of gingerroot with the water, but this would be considered a medicinal tea, not to be drunk every day.

As a spice. Ayurveda recommends a variety of ways to use ginger in cooking. Either the powder or the root can be added to recipes for steamed vegetables, curries, gingerbread, cakes, and cookies. You can *lightly* sprinkle ginger on your food at

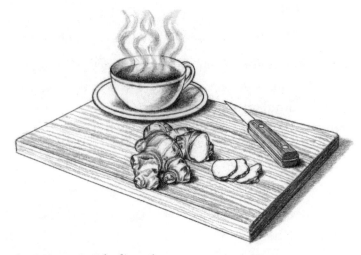

Fresh ginger tea aids digestion.

the table or chew on a sliver of fresh ginger during the meal. Although it may be too strong for everyone, scattering chopped gingerroot over your food as a garnish (like parsley) is also considered worthwhile. Try one approach at a time, however; it does not take much ginger to kindle agni.

Different body types are advised to take ginger in slightly different ways: Vata types can mix the chopped fresh root with salt. Pitta types need less pungency, so weak ginger tea is enough for them, sweetened with sugar to make the ginger less spicy. Kapha types (and anyone who is overweight) want it for eliminating excess Kapha from the system, so they can take a good deal of ginger tea sweetened with honey.

If your appetite and/or digestion become poor as the result of nervousness, stress, or illness, an excellent way to restore it is with the following ginger routine.

Ginger Routine

In a small glass, metal, or ceramic bowl, mash four table-spoons each powdered ginger, brown sugar, and ghee (melted, clarified butter, see page 304). Mix to a uniform consistency, cover, and store in a cool place.

Take a little bit of this ginger mixture every day before breakfast, making sure that you follow it with a good breakfast (hot cereal, grape juice, muffins, and herb tea with cinnamon in it is a good menu). Consume the ginger mixture according to the following schedule.

First day: ½ teaspoon	Sixth day: 2½ teaspoons
Second day: 1 teaspoon	Seventh day: 2 teaspoons
Third day: 1½ teaspoons	Eighth day: 1½ teaspoons
Fourth day: 2 teaspoons	Ninth day: 1 teaspoon
Fifth day: 2½ teaspoons	Tenth day: ½ teaspoon

After finishing the ginger routine, your digestion should be normalized. If you still experience digestive difficulty, see a doctor; at the first sign of digestive cramps and pain, do not attempt this routine—consult a physician instead.

Ginger Follow-up

If you are trying to cure a long-standing Vata imbalance or want to keep your digestion at its peak, taking a little fresh ginger every day is a good idea. It is also considered the best preventive against building up ama through improper digestion.

Cut a thin, nickel-sized slice from the end of a fresh gingerroot, cut off the peel, and chop very fine. Add a few drops of lemon juice and a pinch of salt. Eat this mixture a half-hour before lunch and dinner to stimulate your digestion. If that is incovenient, the mixture can be eaten just before the meal.

GHEE

Ghee, or clarified butter, is prized because it increases agni without simultaneously fueling Pitta. Ghee in fact is considered excellent for balancing Pitta. Kapha types generally need to avoid too much oil of any kind, but ghee is the best for them, too. Ghee is used:

As a cooking oil. Small amounts of ghee are good for sautéing vegetables (not for deep-frying). Ghee does not work as well as butter in baking—breads and desserts need the moisture and milk solids in regular butter.

As a flavoring in place of butter. Since ghee is a prepared food, using butter is not the same as using ghee. Where you would ordinarily butter a vegetable dish or a baked potato or mix it into your oatmeal, ghee is a better choice.

As a digestive. Drizzle a teaspoon of ghee over food at the table (more is not better, since too much oil of any type is not healthy).

How to Make Ghee

Place one pound unsalted butter in a one-quart saucepan over low heat. Allow to melt completely, then raise heat to medium. Skim off foam as it rises. When the butter starts to boil, giving off its water content, lower heat again and cook slowly for about ten minutes. The ghee is done when all the moisture has cooked out and the milk solids at the bottom of the pan have turned light golden brown (there will also be a nutty aroma, but no hint of burning). Remove from heat, let cool, and pour into a clean glass jar or bowl. Ghee keeps indefinitely in the refrigerator but can also be stored at cool or even room temperature for several weeks.

OTHER SPICES FOR GOOD AGNI

Herbs and spices can be selected for each body type, as we did in the Vata-, Pitta-, and Kapha-pacifying diets. But certain ones are good for generally improving the quality of agni.

Black pepper	Clove
Cardamom	Horseradish
Cayenne	Mustard
Cinnamon	

(Pitta types have to be careful to use these in small amounts, since they tend to increase Pitta dosha.)

Building up excess Kapha will make digestion difficult by decreasing agni; it is also bad for building up ama, since both are cold, heavy, and viscous. Using bitter and pungent herbs will reduce Kapha and also "scrape" ama out of the tissues. Ayurveda specifically recommends bitter taste for purification. Among the more common spices that attack ama are:

Black pepper	Clove
Cayenne	Ginger
Cinnamon	

As you can see, these are some of the spices recommended for stimulating agni. The regular but moderate use of these flavorings in your cooking will help prevent ama from forming. Chewing fennel seed after a meal and sweetening your herb tea with raw, uncooked honey are also standard practices for balancing agni.

A BLISSFUL DIET

If bliss is basic to life, there should be a physical counterpart for it in the body, and indeed there is. According to Ayurveda, the body's counterpart to pure joy is a subtle substance called *ojas*, which is extracted from food once it has been perfectly digested. Like the doshas, ojas is just on the edge of being physical; one could call it a subtle substance that registers on both mind and body. The final and most valuable result of eating a good diet is to extract every drop of this subtle substance from your food. That enables the cells to "feel happy," to experience the cellular equivalent of bliss.

Twenty years ago, the idea of a happy cell would have made little sense in scientific terms. Now we know that the body in fact is capable of generating a complex network of chemicals (neurotransmitters, neuropeptides, and related molecules) that the brain uses to communicate emotions throughout the body. It is also known that a single meal can change the brain's biochemistry quite radically. A brain chemical connected with feelings of well-being, such as serotonin, goes up and down in response to the food being digested in the intestinal tract. This has opened up the exciting possibility of a "food pharmacy" to correct depression, anxiety, and other mental disorders, just as fiber helps to correct cholesterol.

In Ayurveda we can bypass the bewildering complexity of brain chemistry. Nature has given us ojas, a single substance for happiness that the body makes all the time.

THE SATTVIC DIET

Ideally, any food you eat is turned into ojas. At the breast, a baby naturally turns his mother's milk into ojas, but it would take a remarkable digestive tract to produce ojas from three-day-old leftover pizza. An excellent, balanced diet can be planned around the foods that turn into ojas with the least effort on your body's part. Ayurveda calls these the sattvic, or pure, foods.

Sattvic Diet

Milk	Rice
Ghee (clarified butter)	Sesame, almonds
Fruits and fruit juices	Sweet taste in general

To this list one often sees added wheat, mung beans, coconut, oranges, dates, and honey. You do not need to be compulsive about these few foods, or eat them exclusively. Just include them in your diet on a regular basis. On a more general level, a sattvic diet contains:

- Light, soothing, easily digested food
- Fresh produce
- Spring water
- Balance of all six tastes
- Moderate portions

According to Ayurveda, this is the best diet for physical strength, a good mind, good health, and longevity. It is conducive to happiness and loving emotions because it is in tune with nature as a whole. The list of sattvic foods is short and would not fulfill a normal person's dietary requirements, although if well managed, a diet limited to milk, vegetables, rice, and fruit would certainly be excellent for one's health. The famous Duke University rice diet, based only on boiled rice and fruit, is recognized as an effective therapeutic regime for heart patients, diabetics, and obese people.

Milk is currently unfashionable among health-conscious people, who tend to link it with digestive problems, allergies, and high cholesterol. Ayurveda holds that most of the objections to milk have to do with consuming it improperly. Milk should be boiled before drinking, which makes it more digestible. It can be drunk hot, warm, or cool, but never ice cold, straight out of the refrigerator. Milk should not be taken with tastes that conflict with it (pungent, sour, salty) but only with other sweet foods (such as grains, sweet fruits, and cereals). Whenever possible, drink milk from organic dairies that do not use hormones or pesticides and have a stated commitment to treat their cows compassionately.

Sweet foods aside, it is recommended that you drink milk alone rather than with your meals, since this is easier on your digestive tract. Low-fat milk may be best for Kapha types, but whole milk is preferred for all other body types (unless there is a problem with high cholesterol, in which case skim milk is best). If you still have trouble digesting milk after it is boiled, or if it seems to create mucous congestion, try adding two pinches of either turmeric or dry ginger before boiling (adding a little raw sugar or honey will cut the bitter taste of the turmeric). These measures remove most of the current objections to milk, which Ayurveda traditionally considers an excellent food for bodily strength, longevity, and peace of mind. Cow's milk is favored above others as the most sattvic.

To move in the direction of a more sattvic diet, try having your next plate of pasta with butter, cream, and Parmesan cheese instead of tomato sauce with meat, onions, and garlic. Any such change, even for one or two meals, should amply demonstrate that sattvic eating makes digestion easier, gives you more energy after you eat, and infuses a light, buoyant feeling throughout the body. (If you want to measure this difference accurately, don't drink alcohol with your meals while you are experimenting.) If your cholesterol is elevated, go easy on the butter and cream; tossing the pasta with olive oil, fresh basil, and a touch of Parmesan is a delicious substitute.

Another example of a sattvic food is sweet lassi, an excellent digestive aid that can be drunk during mild or warm weather (it may tend to promote excessive Kapha in the chill of winter).

Sweet Lassi

For four people, place a scant quarter teaspoon of cardamom, a pinch of saffron threads, and three tablespoons of hot water in a blender. Blend for ten seconds. Add two cups plain yogurt, two cups cool water, and two tablespoons sugar; blend until smooth. If your mixture tastes too sharp, add a quarter cup heavy cream. Adding a few drops of rose water at the end is quite sattvic and cools Pitta (rose water is available at Indian and Middle Eastern groceries and many health-food stores).

BITS—BODY INTELLIGENCE TIPS

In Ayurveda, *how* you eat is just as important as *what* you eat. The reason goes back to ojas, which is the end product of all the signals that reach your body during a meal. Although eating food that tastes good is important, the other senses— sight, hearing, touch, and smell—also need to send signals that make your body happy; that is the only way to completely make use of the mind body connection. An attractive plate of food served steaming hot from the kitchen sends all the right signals to nourish the doshas, but if you leave that plate on the table for five hours, it will be unfit to eat, despite the fact that its raw nutrients have not significantly changed.

Your whole body is tremendously alert while you are eating. Your stomach cells are aware of the conversation at the dinner table, and if they hear harsh words, the stomach will knot with distress. Then everything you digest at that meal will be affected, because you have taken in indigestible sounds. Your stomach cells cannot literally hear, but the brain, taking in what the ears hear, sends out chemical messages to update the stomach and every other organ. So you cannot fool any part of your digestive tract into thinking that a tense meal is a happy one; your "gut feelings" know better.

According to Ayurveda, your duty to your body is to nourish every cell in it in every way—that is the larger purpose of a sattvic diet. If you are careful about nourishing your cells completely, they will reward you with ojas, the perfect expression of their satisfaction. To make that happen, I have provided sixteen BITS, or Body Intelligence Tips, each of which helps to expand the satisfaction your body derives from eating.

As you follow these BITS, you will be surprised at how much more enjoyment every meal can give you. Your body can bubble with joy after every breakfast, lunch, and dinner, once you know the secret of turning food into ojas.

BITS—BODY INTELLIGENCE TIPS

1. Eat in a settled atmosphere.
2. Never eat when you are upset.
3. Always sit down to eat.
4. Eat only when you feel hungry.
5. Reduce ice-cold food and drink.
6. Don't talk while chewing your food.
7. Eat at a moderate pace, neither too fast nor too slow.
8. Wait until one meal is digested before eating the next (i.e., intervals of two to four hours for light meals, four to six for full meals).

9. Sip warm water with your meal.
10. Eat freshly cooked meals whenever possible.
11. Minimize raw foods—cooked food (preferably well cooked) is much easier to digest.
12. Do not cook with honey—heated honey is considered to produce ama.
13. Drink milk separately from meals, either alone or with other sweet foods.
14. Experience all six tastes at every meal.
15. Leave one-third to one-quarter of your stomach empty to aid digestion.
16. Sit quietly for a few minutes after your meal.

This concise list gives you a great head start on getting the most out of any diet. The basic principle here is that food that is easiest to digest is best for you, which explains why well-cooked food is preferred over raw, hot over cold, fresh over processed. Making digestion easier is also the reason for sipping warm water with your meal, eliminating milk, and sitting briefly at the table once you are finished eating in order for your body to settle into its digestive rhythms.

Another important principle is moderation. Moderate amounts of food are taken at regular mealtimes—the Ayurvedic texts consider a double handful of food to be an ideal portion. Take this amount as a first serving and go back for more if you still feel hungry. It is advisable to leave one-third to one-quarter of your stomach empty at the end of your meal. Your digestive tract will work more efficiently on smaller portions, and your body will find it much easier to control its weight automatically. Don't be afraid that you will walk away from the table hungry. Being satisfied is not the same as being stuffed. If you leave a little empty room in your stomach, you will feel light, buoyant, energetic, and much fresher an hour after you eat. That is how a properly eaten meal feels, leading naturally to a properly digested one.

BITS for Weight Loss

If you have a problem with overweight, try using these BITS before going on any kind of calorie-cutting diet. You will be surprised to find that your excess weight is caused not just by what you've been eating but by how you've been eating it—carelessly or compulsively, on the run instead of sitting down, between meals instead of at regular hours. These are simple things, of course, but they make a big difference.

Leaving aside the very small minority who actually have a hormone or metabolic problem, most overweight people are the victims of conditioning—bad habits that have been unconsciously built into their bodies over time. Everyone's body has the intelligence to know the right amount to eat; nature gave us the hunger reflex to tell us when our bodies want food and its opposite, the satiation reflex, to tell us when our stomachs are satisfied. People who have lost these instincts have surrendered an important aspect of their body's intelligence. They eat like machines, switched on by automatic cues—the sight and smell of food, or just the thought of it. But by following these BITS they can return to "conscious eating," guided by their body's inner intelligence.

WHEN OJAS IS LESS

Besides overeating, other abuses at the table can suppress our healthy instincts for eating. If you consume a meal while feeling angry, an Ayurvedic doctor would say that you are producing mental ama from your food, while a Western physician would say that a stress reaction is throwing off your endocrine balance. The end result is the same, a damaging chemical message going straight to your cells.

Even before you eat the first bite of food, disturbances in the doshas can negate your body's attempt to produce ojas. As usual, Vata dosha comes into play here—whatever throws off Vata dosha also damages ojas—worry, loud noise, going without sleep, and drastic diets and fasting. On the positive side, anything that calms Vata during mealtimes is good for ojas.

Most people do not eat a strictly sattvic diet in this country, so I would like to give a few more reasons why changing to one would benefit your health. You will notice that a sattvic diet is vegetarian, and it is now common knowledge that vegetarians have excellent blood pressure (18 percent lower than average) and lower rates of heart disease and cancer. In addition, the federal government has warned us for twenty-five years that Americans eat far too much salt, protein, and animal fat, most of which comes from meat (much of the excess salt also comes from processed foods). If you started reducing your meat intake today, moving gradually in the direction of a meatless diet, you would almost certainly lessen your chance of having a heart attack in the future. By including sweet foods on the list, Ayurveda does not mean to condone the huge amounts of refined white sugar that most of us now consume. The sweetness of pasta, rice, and bread is enough.

Like everything else, there are two extremes in diet. Certain foods are not easily turned into ojas; among them are the following:

Non-Ojas Diet

- Meat, poultry, and fish
- Heavy and oily foods
- Cheese

- Leftovers and processed food
- Excess of sour, salty tastes
- Overeating

For the sake of economy and convenience, many cooks like to save leftovers, but Ayurveda frowns on this practice. Food is meant to be eaten fresh, right off the stove if not right out of the garden—the fresher the produce, the more the ojas. Old, cold food, even when reheated, will not produce ojas in the same amounts. Frozen food in general is also good to avoid. Drinking alcohol and smoking cigarettes destroys ojas and prevents other foods from producing it. Air and water pollution are equally detrimental. All of these influences are called tamasic, which means that they produce dullness and inertia by promoting the buildup of ama. Kapha types should be especially wary, since their naturally slow digestion makes it easier for ama to form.

Finally, here are a few time-honored rules about a blissful diet handed down in the Ayurvedic tradition, each aimed at maximizing ojas.

- Eat fresh food suitable to the season and your geographical area. The best possible foods for the body are fruits, vegetables, and dairy products raised in your area—foods have thrived on the same air, water, nutrients, and sunlight that you grow on.
- Have your largest meal at lunch, when digestion is strongest. Dinner should be a modest meal that can be digested before bedtime; breakfast is optional and in any case should be your smallest meal of the day.
- Eat at the same time every day. Besides not snacking, avoid eating at night, which disturbs your digestive

rhythms and easily promotes ama as you sleep from the food that is undigested.

- Dine either alone or with people you genuinely like. Negative emotions, whether yours, the cook's, or those of the people around you, have a harmful effect on digestion.
- Be grateful for nature's unending gift of food, and respect it as you do yourself.

CHAPTER 13

EXERCISE—THE MYTH OF "NO PAIN, NO GAIN"

From an Ayurvedic standpoint, much of the exercise recommended today falls short of ideal. Why do we need physical activity in the first place? Charaka, the greatest writer on Ayurveda, gave this answer: "From physical exercise one gets lightness, a capacity for work, firmness, tolerance of difficulties, elimination of impurities, and stimulation of digestion." Aerobics for your heart or weight training for your muscles achieve some of these goals, but these are not comprehensive enough activities to fit Charaka's description. The ideal is to balance the whole system, mind and body. It is also vital that exercise give more energy than it takes, a consideration that people tend to ignore.

One very simple exercise, walking, comes close to being ideal because it is a natural activity that satisfies all three doshas. Vata types find that taking a long walk tranquilizes them. Pitta types react quite differently. They like being slowed down from the driving pace that so often overtakes them during their workday. Kaphas feel stimulated and lighter; a brisk walk clears out any minor congestion they might have built up and makes their typically slow digestion more efficient. For these reasons, a brisk half-hour walk every day is one of the prime recommendations we make to patients at the Chopra Center.

Patients are also taught a new approach to exercise in which the aim is not to strain or to pound their muscles into shape. They are shown that exercise is meant to forge a closer link between themselves and their quantum mechanical bodies—it thus becomes a powerful tool for balance. We call this approach "three-dosha exercise." It is embodied in a set of short, connected routines:

- The Sun Salute (*Surya Namaskara*)—a morning exercise that combines stretching, balance, and calisthenics (1 to 6 minutes)
- Neuromuscular integration—a set of gentle yoga positions (10 to 15 minutes)
- Balanced breathing—a simple form of *Pranayama*, a traditional yogic breath exercise (5 minutes)

The description of these exercises begins on page 325. Performing them in connection with meditation, for which they are ideally suited, raises mind body integration to a new level. To begin with, these exercises are natural and comfortable forms of activity that the doshas welcome. They can also be performed by all age groups and do not require you to be in shape.

From the very first session, people discover the intimacy that nature has established between awareness and physiology. The body is not just a shell or a walking life-support system. It is your self intimately clothed in matter. Getting back in touch with this intimacy is very reassuring and delightful, particularly for people who have given up on exercise and become virtual strangers to their bodies.

SUCCESS WITHOUT PAIN

Before explaining these points further, let's consider conventional exercise. Since life is generally meant to be comfortable and happy, Ayurveda views exercise as a means to that end. It holds that exercise should always leave you ready for work. Exercise shouldn't be work itself. Yet, many Americans see it that way. They feel that without a grim and determined attitude, they are not doing much good for themselves. (Go to the park early tomorrow morning and count how many frowns there are on the faces of the runners you see.) If you get only one benefit from Ayurveda's approach to exercise, it should be that "no pain, no gain" is a myth.

A good way to see this is in terms of Vata dosha. All physical activity increases Vata. A moderate increase makes you feel more vigorous, alert, and clearheaded, as well as stronger physically. You are getting mental and physical benefits together, in a natural balance. But overstimulating Vata destroys all these benefits. It makes you feel restless, fatigued, and shaky.

How much is enough, then? As a general rule, Ayurveda wants us to exercise to 50 percent of maximum capacity. If you can bicycle ten miles, go for five; if you can swim twenty laps, make it ten. These lower limits are not detrimental to fitness; in fact they make exercise more efficient, because you are not giving your body so much repair work to do afterward, and your cardiovascular system will have an easier time returning to normal after your workout. Another simple guideline has to do with exertion. Rather than exerting yourself to the point where you are sweating heavily and panting for breath, just go until you break out into a light sweat and start to mouth breathe. Those are natural signals that you are at the right limit.

You are going too far if you begin to pant or sweat profusely, if you feel your heart pounding violently, or if your knees feel rubbery. At the first sign of overexertion, stop exercising, give yourself a few minutes of walking around to let the system cool down by stages, and then rest for another few minutes until your pulse and breathing are back to normal. In the heat of competitive sports such as tennis and racquetball, you may not notice how strenuously you are exerting yourself. If it is fun to play, then keep on. But if you are pushing yourself to win the game or to prove that you can keep up with someone else, your attitude is needlessly punishing your body.

Vata types especially should be careful not to overdo; their constitutions generally have lower exercise thresholds than Pittas, and Pittas lower than Kaphas. Exertion also needs to be adjusted for age: over the age of 45 or 50, everyone begins to have increased Vata, which should be compensated for by not exercising as hard as before. As in everything else, you need to respect your doshas. Going the extra mile at any age is just another way of inviting serious Vata problems. (Recent studies in sports medicine indicate that 50 percent of serious women athletes have significant menstrual disturbances, a symptom of highly aggravated Vata.)

BODY-TYPE EXERCISE

Every time you move your body, you are talking to your doshas. Because each dosha has its own emphasis, there are three kinds of benefits that all balanced exercise brings:

Vata: poise, agility, limberness, coordination, and inner exhilaration

Pitta: warming up the body, circulation of blood to all parts, increased heart capacity

Kapha: increased strength and stability, steady energy

If you never get out of your armchair to exercise, obviously you will not experience these benefits. But many active people with firm muscles and sound hearts do not experience them either. Most exercise programs today are dedicated to increasing the capacity of the cardiovascular system, which puts a heavy emphasis on Pitta dosha. I would like to list balanced activities that are broader in scope and more suited to the major body types.

VATA-TYPE EXERCISE

Type: Yoga   Amount: Light
      Dance aerobics
      Walking, short hikes
      Light bicycling

Vata types have bursts of energy but tire quickly. They excel at balancing and stretching exercises. Being light and lithe, they like yoga and walking, as long as these do not become too tiring. Because of their natural enthusiasm, Vata types also feel good doing bouncy dance aerobics to music. Any exercise that takes place indoors is good in winter, since Vata people are averse to the cold and do not have enough fat and muscle to protect them from the elements.

Everyone dominated by Vata must always be careful not to get carried away and push themselves too far. This is the primary caution for them, since Vata dosha typically starts with a bang but does not know its limits, particularly when out of balance. Half an hour of mild exercise a day is enough. If you are exhausted, trembling, dizzy, or on the verge of cramping, you have gone much too far. These are all signs of Vata imbalance.

PITTA-TYPE EXERCISE

Type: Skiing   Amount: Moderate
     Brisk walking or jogging
     Hiking and mountain climbing
     Swimming

Pitta types tend to have more drive than endurance. They are good at all exercise in moderation. Because they like a challenge above all, Pittas enjoy skiing, hiking, mountain climbing, and other sports that bring a sense of accomplishment at the end of the day.

Athletes in competitive sports must have a good deal of Pitta to give them a fighting spirit, but this is not the dosha for intense competition. Pittas hate to lose; this motivates them more than the satisfaction of winning. (Sports studies have shown this among professional tennis players, some of whom are notorious for Pitta-type anger.) Pittas will grimly make themselves run, jog, or weight train but gain very little inner contentment from their efforts.

Probably you already know whether you are falling into this trap. If you stew over every bad shot on the golf course or want to drill your tennis opponent with the ball, give up these sports. If you chew yourself or anyone else out in any sport, walk away from it. Anyone who needs to kill somebody on the court is suffering from gross Pitta imbalance. Also, the start-stop rhythm of competition sports is not as good for your body as half an hour of continuous motion.

Walking briskly for half an hour a day will take the feistiness out of your system better than a competitive sport.

Swimming is even better—many Pitta types who drive themselves on the job find that a plunge in the pool at five o'clock cools them off and dissolves the day's tensions. Winter sports of all kinds also appeal to Pittas because they take to the cold better than Vata and Kapha types. Because they are stimulated visually, Pittas gain a large benefit from a leisurely stroll in the woods; it provides a change from their usual determined pace. The beauty of nature will sink deep into them when they pause long enough to experience it.

KAPHA-TYPE EXERCISE

Type: Weight training   Amount: Moderately heavy
  Running
  Aerobics
  Rowing
  Dance

Kapha types have strong, steady energy but often lack agility. They generally are good at all exercises and become better when they become more limber and balanced. Because of their physical strength, Kaphas excel at endurance sports—they have the natural build for a long run or distance rowing. The combination of Pitta and Kapha gives determination and endurance. This is a common prakruti among professional baseball and football players.

Pushing the blood through their veins feels good to Kaphas, which is why they take to weight training in gyms and health clubs. It is good to combine this with exercise that gets the circulation going; bringing up a good sweat (without exhaustion) will clear out Kapha congestion. Many Kaphas have excess fat and water that need to be pushed out. Being a cold dosha, Kapha resents it if you go out into the cold and damp to run or row. In winter, Kapha types should stay indoors and stick with aerobics or calisthenics.

Dance classes provide a good alternative for Kaphas. Although a Kapha may not have a dancer's build, they feel much better about their natural shape, once they gain the poise and balance that dance training instills.

A few general precautions apply to all body types. Do not exercise:

- *Just before or after a meal.* Exercising at these times lowers your agni, which you want at its highest. Allow at least half an hour before a meal and one to two hours afterward without exercising. Walking right after a meal, however, is an exception. Taking a leisurely fifteen-minute walk after lunch and/or dinner stimulates digestion (anything longer or harder would compete with it). Exercising after sundown is discouraged by Ayurveda; it is better to let your body slow down in the evening and prepare itself for bed.
- *In the wind or the cold.* Both Vata and Kapha dosha resent the cold, as we have mentioned. If you go out for a walk in winter, keep yourself bundled up and do not breathe strenuously. Heavy breathing of cold, damp air is bad for the respiratory tract. Also, any strong wind upsets Vata dosha and removes the calming effect of a good walk.

- *In the broiling sun.* The reason only mad dogs and Englishmen go out in the noonday sun is that harsh sun inflames Pitta dosha, raising your body heat at a time when exercise is raising it enough already.

Along with moderation, the key to balanced exercise is regularity. The doshas always tend to reinforce themselves. If you have neglected physical activity for a while, your body will be used to inertia. Once you return to even a little activity, your doshas will rise to a level of better balance and want to stay there. So, do everything you can to start a program that you will enjoy for years, preferably for life.

THREE-DOSHA EXERCISES

Now I would like to describe the three-dosha exercises taught at our Center: the Sun Salute, the set of gentle yoga positions, and balanced breathing. More people in the West are becoming familiar with these postures and discovering the benefits that have been appreciated in the East for thousands of years.

The following exercises are very easy to do. Only the Sun Salute requires some patience to master; the others do not take any special skill. The whole emphasis on perfect performance is misplaced. These are exercises for tuning in to your body. Anyone can do that, simply by letting the mind relax into each pose. Don't even think of how you look or how close you are coming to the ideal positions. Whatever you achieve is right for you. This approach makes each exercise feel good as you do it and even better afterward. Everyone feels pleasantly relaxed for the next few hours after doing a short Ayurvedic routine.

The following descriptions were provided by Bija Bennett, an expert, talented yoga therapist who has taught yoga at many of our seminars over the years.

SUN SALUTE *(Surya Namaskara)*

Time: 1 to 2 minutes for each cycle, moving slowly
Repetitions: 1 to 6 cycles in the morning, more as you
  become experienced

The Sun Salute *(Surya Namaskara)* is a complete Ayurvedic exercise that simultaneously integrates the whole physiology—mind, body, and breath. It strengthens and stretches all the major muscle groups, lubricates the joints, conditions the spine, and massages the internal organs. Blood flow and circulation is increased throughout the body. With regular practice, you will gain stability, suppleness, flexibility, and grace.

Here is a cycle of 12 postures. Perform them in a fluid sequence one right after another. Synchronize each motion with the breath. Move smoothly into each pose, breathing fully and easily so that each cycle takes about 1 minute.

Start slowly, avoiding strain, and listen to your body as you gradually increase the number of Sun Salute cycles you do. This step-by-step progression eliminates the possibility of pulling or tiring your muscles, especially if you haven't been exercising regularly. Stop when you notice that you are breathing and perspiring heavily or feeling too tired. If this occurs, lie down and rest for a minute or two until the breath is free. With regular performance, your capacity will easily and naturally increase.

In the Sun Salute, a specific pattern of breathing is encouraged. Inhale to extend your spine vertically or to open, lengthen, or fully elongate the body. Exhale to bend or fold the body, creating a flexing of the spine. Each of your movements should be an extension of the breath in order to facilitate the motion. There is one transitional position in the Sun Salute where the breath pauses for a moment before you continue into the next pose. Otherwise, let your breathing be fluid and continuous throughout the entire exercise.

HOW TO PERFORM THE SUN SALUTE

Perform the following postures in a flowing, moving sequence one right after another. Remember to use the breath to connect each pose with the one following it. Emphasize the expansion of the chest on inhale and the contraction of the abdomen or belly in a bending motion on exhale.

1. Salutation position (*Samasthiti*). Begin by standing tall with the feet together in a parallel position. Stand evenly on both feet and lengthen the spine upward. Place the palms of your hands together in front of your chest. Lift the chest and expand the ribs as you look straight ahead.

2. Raised arm position (*Tadasana*). On the inhalation, slowly extend the arms over the head. Lift and expand the chest as you continue lengthening the spine while allowing the head to look upward. Keep breathing evenly as you continue right into the next pose.

3. Hand to foot position (*Uttanasana*). As you exhale, bend the body forward and down, lengthening the spine, arms, and neck. Let the knees soften or bend freely, bringing the hands to the floor. Avoid collapsing the chest or overrounding the upper back. Keep the elbows and shoulders relaxed, and don't lock the knees.

4. Equestrian position (*Ashwa Sanchalanasana*). On your next inhalation, extend the left leg back and drop the back knee to the ground. The front knee is bent and the supporting

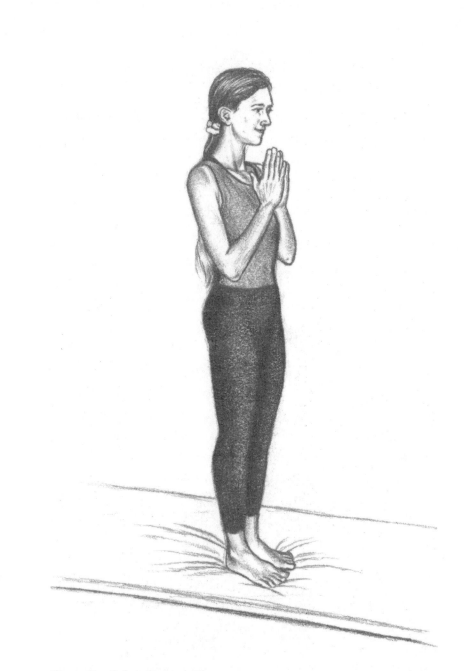

Figure 1.   Salutation position.

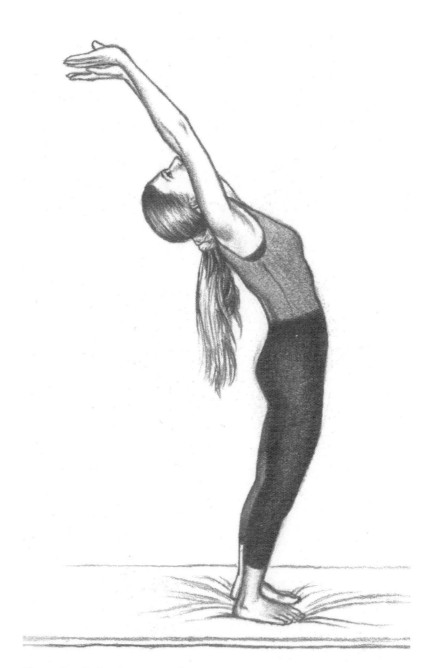

Figure 2. Raised arm position.

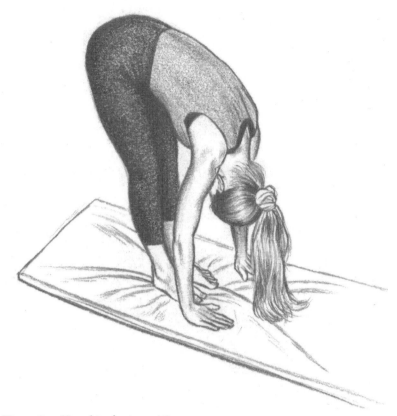

Figure 3.   Hand to foot position.

foot remains flat on the floor. Simultaneously extend or lift the spine and open the chest. Allow the head and neck to lengthen vertically.

5. Mountain position (*Adhomukha Svanasana*). On the exhalation, bring the left leg back to meet the right leg—legs both at hip width apart, hands at shoulder distance. As you raise the buttocks and hips, press down with the hands, allowing the spine to release upward and back. Stretch the heels down toward the floor and lengthen through the backs of the legs. Relax and free the head and neck. The body forms an

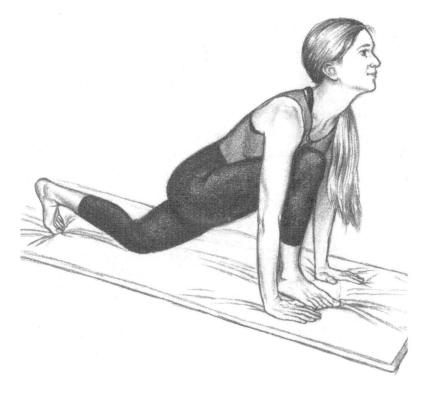

Figure 4. Equestrian position.

even inverted V from the pelvis to the hands and from the pelvis to the heels.

6. Eight limbs position (*Ashtanga Namaskara*). Gently drop both knees to the ground and slowly slide the body down at an angle as you bring the chest and chin to the ground. All eight limbs—both the toes, knees, chest, hands, and chin—touch the floor. Hold this very briefly and then continue to move into the next pose.

7. Cobra position (*Bhujangasana*). On the inhalation, lift and expand the chest forward and up as you press down with

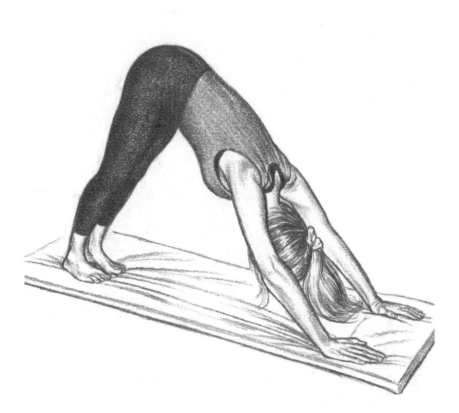

Figure 5. Mountain position.

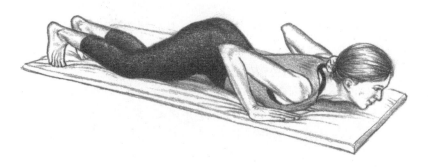

Figure 6. Eight limbs position.

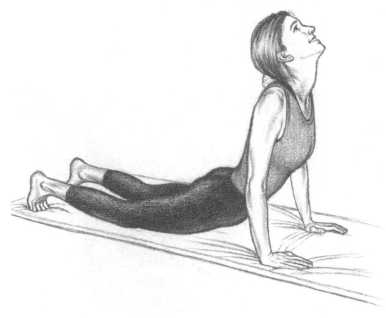

Figure 7.   Cobra position.

the hands. Keep the elbows close to the body and continue to extend the spine upward. Open and widen the chest and move the shoulders down and away from the ears to free the neck and head. Let the upper back widen and lengthen. Do not initiate this movement with the head or lift the body with the neck.

8. Mountain position (*Adhomukha Svanasana*). Repeat position 5. On the exhalation, raise the buttocks and hips, press down with the hands, and allow the spine to release upward and back. Stretch the heels down toward the floor and lengthen through the backs of the legs. Relax and free the head and neck.

9. Equestrian position (*Ashwa Sanchalanasana*). Repeat position 4. Inhale and swing the right leg forward between the hands. The left leg stays extended back, knee to the ground.

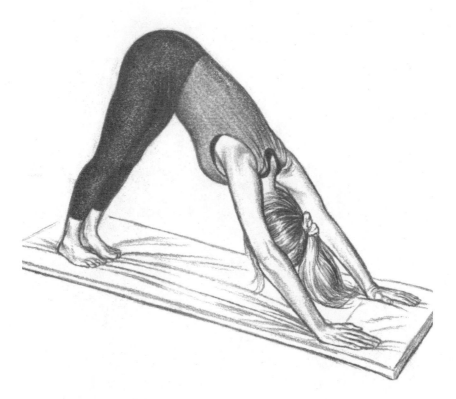

Figure 8. Mountain position.

The front knee should be bent with the foot flat on the floor. Extend the spine, lifting the chest forward and up. Allow the head and neck to lengthen upward.

10. Hand to foot position (*Uttanasana*). Repeat position 3. As you exhale, step forward with the left leg and continue to bend the body forward and down, lengthening the entire spine. The arms and head follow in line with the spine. Both hands remain on the floor. Let the knees soften or bend freely. Avoid collapsing the chest or overrounding the upper back. Keep the elbows and shoulders relaxed.

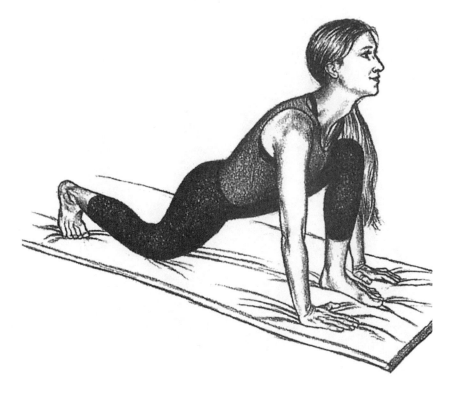

Figure 9. Equestrian position.

11. Raised arm position (*Tadasana*). Repeat position 2. On the inhalation lift the arms from the upper back as you open the chest forward and up. Do not lift the body from the head or neck. Continue to lift and expand the chest as you come up, extending the arms over the head. Keep the breathing smooth, deep, and continuous.

12. Salutation position (*Samasthiti*). Repeat position 1. Exhale as you lower the arms and bring the palms of your hands together in front of your chest. You are standing tall with the feet in a parallel position at hip distance. Lift the chest

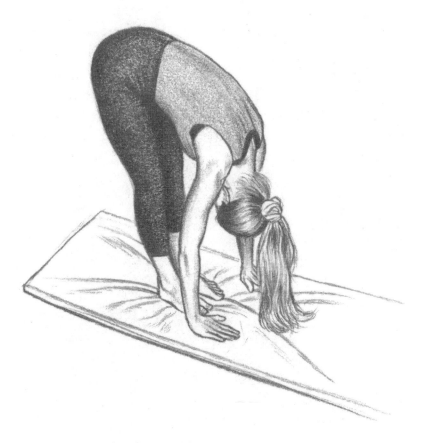

Figure 10. Hand to foot position.

and expand the ribs as you look straight ahead. Vertically lengthen the spine and neck.

This completes one cycle of the Sun Salute.

Hold the Salutation position while continuing to breathe for a few breaths. Then begin the second cycle. This standing Salutation position becomes position 1 of the second set. On the next inhalation, continue into position 2—the raised arm position—and repeat the movements in a fluid sequence.

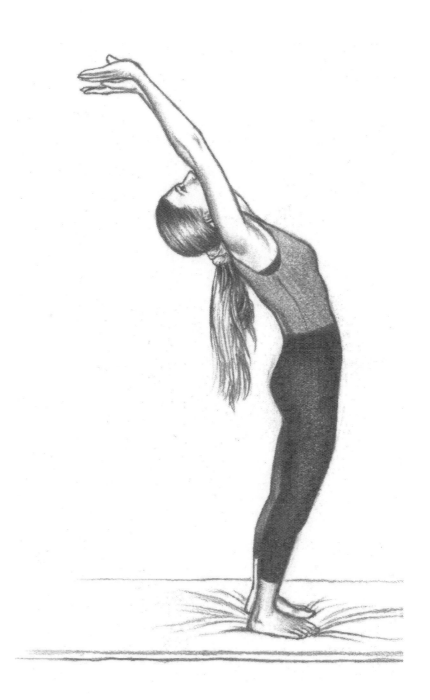

Figure 11.   Raised arm position.

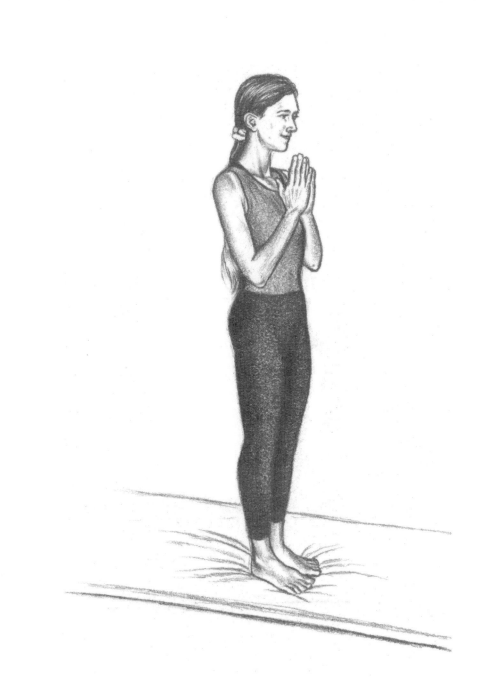

Figure 12.   Salutation position.

On subsequent sets of the Sun Salute, you will alternate which foot is extended back and which swings forward in positions 4 and 9—the Equestrian position. In the first cycle, the left foot extends back in positions 4 and 9, with the right foot forward. Alternate which leg extends back on the next set and continue to alternate sides with each new cycle.

After you have completed the sequence of Sun Salutes, lie on your back, lengthen the spine, and let the body completely relax. Close your eyes and rest for a minute or two. Allow your breath to be free and easy.

YOGA POSITIONS

Time: 10 to 15 minutes, moving slowly
Repetitions: 1 set in the morning and 1 set in the afternoon

The following easy poses, which take about 15 minutes to perform, are considered the basic Ayurvedic exercise. A set can be practiced before morning and afternoon meditation, with or without the Sun Salute. These positions are taught as part of the neuromuscular integration program at our Center and are comfortable for anyone in good health, regardless of age or previous physical training.

What follows is a specific sequence that begins with toning and warming up the body. The set continues with seated and forward bends, standing postures, inverted poses, backbending postures, twists, a resting pose, and ends with a short breathing exercise. Each of the postures in this sequence has a specific therapeutic effect on the physiology. We will mention a few of the well-known benefits of each pose, as given in the ancient texts.

In general, the toning and warm-up exercises increase circulation and improve blood flow to the entire body. Seated poses help to create stability, proper spinal alignment, and good posture, while the forward bends stimulate digestion, increase the spine's flexibility, and calm the physiology. Backbends create mobility and suppleness in the spine—especially in the upper back—and at the same time are invigorating. Inverted poses stimulate the endocrine system and allow for increased circulation, while twists aid digestion, elimination, and tone the spinal column. All of these postures are succeeded by the resting pose and breathing exercises, which bring increased awareness, orderliness, and balance.

A sequence of postures is important because it first prepares the body in order to warm it up and remove stiffness. It progresses to invigorate, strengthen, and stretch the entire body. This is why it is valuable to practice in an orderly sequence, as each pose is a preparation for the following posture or a counterbalance for the preceding one.

Here are a few guidelines to follow before practicing:

Perform the postures slowly, making sure you inhale and exhale, without holding the breath or controlling it in any way. Breathing should be easy, fluid, and continuous.

1. No pain, most gain. If you can't touch your toes without excruciating effort, do not push. Let the knees soften or bend freely. **Never strain or push the body in these exercises.** Hold the postures for a few seconds and then release easily. Movements should be performed slowly and comfortably. Never move in or out of the postures abruptly or bounce in a pose. Use the breath to facilitate the movement.

2. How far should you reach? In each pose, go to the point where you feel the stretch. Just move as far as you easily can

without effort. Allow your awareness to naturally go to the area of the body that is being stretched. Don't overextend, force, or overstretch. Sometimes it helps to release or back off completely from the stretch, then easily stretch it again. *Do not forget to breathe!*

3. Over the months you'll notice increased strength, flexibility, and suppleness. So it is not necessary to push the body to reach a desired goal. In fact, these postures are not designed to impose a specific structure on your body, and there is no "ideal" pose. Rather, your progress comes from the integrated functioning of awareness, movement, and breath.

4. All Ayurvedic exercise involves the mind as well as the body. In each exercise, a particular area is stretched. Allow your awareness to naturally go to that area. The softening of the accumulated stress is said to come from letting the attention be on the area of stretch.

For that reason, allow the exercises to have your full attention. Don't play the radio or TV in the background. Just let your mind be easily aware of your body.

5. Wear comfortable, loose clothing. Use a flat, nonslippery surface, but avoid performing these exercises on a bare floor. Rather, use a folded wool blanket, rug, exercise mat, or other semisoft surface.

6. *Note:* It is important to mention that all postures should be adapted to meet the needs of the individual. In certain situations, such as acute illness, pregnancy, menstruation, and specific structural problems, the posture may be adjusted or changed in order to be more effective and to serve one's particular requirement. In any of these special cases, please check with a qualified yoga instructor.

I. TONING-UP EXERCISES (1 to 2 minutes)

We begin with a few exercises that invigorate and tone the body. The first exercise consists of progressively massaging the body with the hands and fingers, moving in the direction of the heart.

1. First come to a comfortable sitting position. Using the palms and fingers of both hands, press the top of your head and gradually continue to press and release with the hands moving forward over the face and down the neck and chest. Again start at the top of the head and press the head with the palms and fingers moving down and over the back of the neck, coming around to the chest.

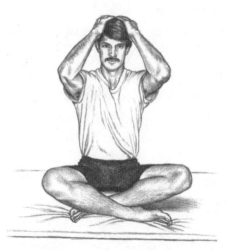

Figure 1. Toning-up exercise, head.

2. To tone the hands and arms, begin by massaging the right side first. Grasp the fingers of the right hand with your left hand and continue to press and release upward along the top of the right arm all the way to the shoulder and across the

chest. Repeat by pressing and releasing along the underside of the right arm, from the hand up to the forearm, shoulder, and chest. Your pressure should be firm and the massage should be gradual and continuous. Repeat on the left side, making sure to massage both the top and underside of the arm.

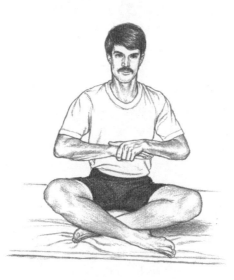

Figure 2.   Toning-up exercise, hands.

3. Bring the tips of the fingers to your navel and with both hands on the belly, begin to press and release around the abdomen, gradually moving the pressure up to the heart.

4. Massage by pressing and releasing your lower back, kidney area, and ribs, moving up toward the heart.

5. Start with the right foot, grasping and massaging the toes, soles, and tops of the feet, moving up the calves, thighs, hips, and stomach, continuing the motion up toward the heart. Repeat on the left leg, moving up to the hips and continuing all the way to the heart.

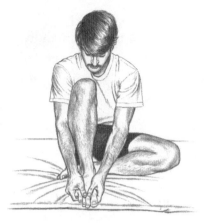

Figure 3.   Toning-up exercise, feet.

6. Lie on your back and lengthen the spine, keeping the head and neck long and free. Bring the knees up to your chest, clasp your hands over the knees, and begin to roll slowly and easily from side to side. Always allow your neck to be relaxed and free. Breathe normally.

7. Roll 5 times to each side and then release the arms and slowly extend your legs out from the hips. Let the body be completely relaxed.

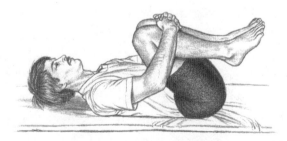

Figure 4.   Toning-up exercise, side roll.

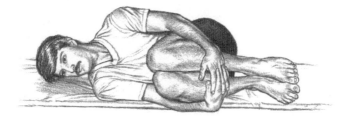

Figure 5. Toning-up exercise, side roll.

II. SEAT FIRMING POSE—*Vajrasana* (30 seconds to 1 minute)

1. Begin by kneeling and sitting with the buttocks on the heels. The feet should be slightly apart and the big toes crossed. Lengthen the spine, widen the rib cage, and slightly lift the chest. The head and neck should be long and free. Look straight ahead and breathe easily. Place your hands in your lap with the right hand on top of the left, palms up.

2. As you inhale, lift the buttocks off the heels and come up to a kneeling position. Keep the spine lengthened and the chest open and lifted. Relax the shoulders. On the exhalation, slowly lower the body and sit back down on the heels. Repeat again smoothly, with even breaths.

3. Move slowly. Breathe deeply and easily, keeping the front and back of your body lively, long, and free.

Benefits: This asana strengthens the pelvic region, removes tension from the knees and ankles, and builds a strong foundation for the back.

III. HEAD TO KNEE POSE—*Janu Sírsasana*
(About 1 minute)

1. Sit down and extend your legs straight out in front of you. Stretch through the backs of the legs and heels, toes pointing up toward the head.

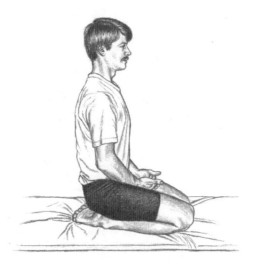

Figure 6.   Seat-firming pose, starting position.

2. Bend your left knee and place the sole of your left foot against the inside of the right thigh.

3. Inhale and lift your arms straight up from the upper back, stretching them over your head. On the exhalation, bend your body forward and down, elongating the spine. Keep lengthening the spine, arms, and neck as you come forward. Avoid collapsing your chest or overrounding your upper back. You may soften the front knee slightly to further release your lower back.

4. Hold the pose for a few breaths. Then inhale and release your arms from the upper back, opening the chest forward

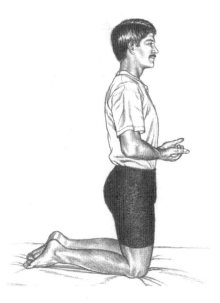

Figure 7.   Seat-firming pose, erect position.

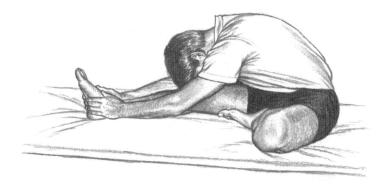

Figure 8.   Head to knee pose.

and up as you bring your arms over the head. Repeat again on the same side, moving slowly and comfortably. Inhale as you raise your body and exhale as you lower your arms down to your sides.

5. Perform this posture on the other side. Fully extend your left leg in front of you. Bend your right knee and place the sole of your right foot against the inside of your left thigh.

6. Breathe and move into the posture slowly. Exhale as you bend your body forward and down and inhale as you come up. Then repeat the pose again on the same side. Breathe normally and hold for a few breaths without strain. After you come up, exhale and lower your arms down to the sides.

Benefits: This pose strengthens and relaxes the spine, tones the abdomen, liver, and spleen, and aids in digestion.

IV. SHOULDER STAND—*Sarvangasana* (Start by holding for 30 seconds; gradually increase to 2 minutes if you are comfortable in the pose.)

Note of Caution: If you are a beginner or have stiffness or problems in the upper back and neck, practice this posture with one or two blankets placed under the shoulders to protect the neck, or do a half shoulder stand rather than completely straightening the body in the full pose. Perform this posture slowly. If you have a chronic back problem or high blood pressure, be sure to check with your doctor before performing this pose. (Ayurveda advises against standing on the head, as it can injure the brain, neck, and spine if practiced improperly.)

1. Lie on your back and press your arms and hands flat against the floor. Relax your shoulders and lengthen the spine.

2. As you exhale, bend your knees and slowly raise your

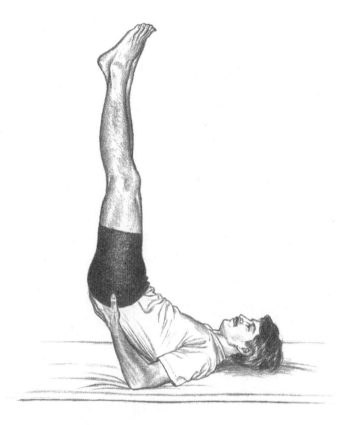

Figure 9.   Shoulder stand.

legs over the waist. Push your palms against the floor and swing your knees up and over your head. Bend the elbows, keeping them in toward the body and in line with your shoulders. Support your back with your hands above the hips. The elbows and the shoulders should create a stable platform to support your body.

3. Straighten your legs by lengthening through both heels and the balls of your feet. Allow your spine to stretch up toward the ceiling. Fully stretch your legs out from the hips to

keep your body in a straight line from the ankles to the shoulders. Extend the spine upward.

4. If you choose to do the half shoulder stand, don't straighten your body all the way. Support the weight of your body with your hands, while making an angle with your legs. The feet point in the direction of the head. (*Note*: This is a shoulder stand, *not* a neck stand, so there should be no strain in the neck or throat. This is very important.) Keep the breath smooth and let your face relax. Hold the posture for a few breaths, increasing the time you stay in this pose as is comfortable.

Benefits: This asana enlivens the entire endocrine system, increases circulation to the thyroid gland, relieves mental fatigue, brings flexibility to the spine, and has a soothing effect on the body.

V. PLOW POSE—*Halasana* (15 seconds to 1 minute)

1. Continue into this next posture as you exhale and bend from the pelvis to bring both legs down over the head. Keep the legs stretching straight out through the heels so that the legs are at a right angle to the torso. Let the spine lengthen to avoid overcurving the upper back. Keep your breath smooth and continuous.

2. Allow your legs to go back only as far as you feel comfortable, without collapsing the spine or chest. Be careful not to put too much strain on the neck. (If you feel pain, slowly release and come out of the pose.)

3. Now extend the arms straight out behind you in the opposite direction, away from your legs and head. The torso should rest on the tops of the shoulders, the hips maintaining a vertical line with the shoulder joints. Lengthen your spine.

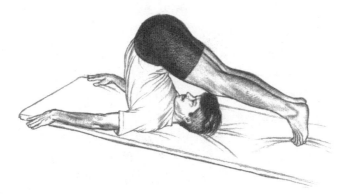

Figure 10. Plow pose, arms extended.

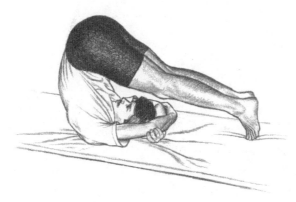

Figure 11. Plow pose, arms behind head.

4. Fold the arms over your head and hold for a few breaths.

5. To come down, exhale, bend your knees, and support the lower back with your hands. Slowly and easily uncurl the spine with the knees bent until you are lying flat. Rest comfortably for a few moments.

6. Be sure to let your breathing be smooth, especially in the Shoulder Stand and Plow. The quality of your breath will be an indication of whether you are straining or pushing too far.

Benefits: The Plow pose strengthens and relaxes the back, neck, and shoulders. It improves performance of the liver and spleen and removes fatigue. Both the Shoulder Stand and the Plow stimulate and normalize functioning of the thyroid gland.

VI. COBRA POSE—*Bhujangasana* (30 seconds to 1 minute)

1. Lie facedown on your stomach, bring the feet together and the hands directly under your shoulders, fingers pointing forward. Slightly elongate the spine to protect your lower back.

2. On the inhalation, lift and expand the chest forward and up as you press down with the hands. Keep your elbows close in to the body and continue to extend the spine upward. Open and widen the chest and move the shoulders down and away from your ears to free the neck and head. Let the upper back widen and lengthen.

3. Hold for a few breaths, then exhale and come down slowly.

4. Repeat the pose 1 to 3 times, beginning with the inhalation and lifting from the chest. Be careful not to initiate this movement from your head or lift the body with your neck. Keep the spine long and breathe normally. Allow your breath to be fluid and easy. Exhale and slowly come down. Let the body relax completely.

Benefits: This pose strengthens the back, stretches the abdominal muscles, and is helpful with uterine and ovarian problems.

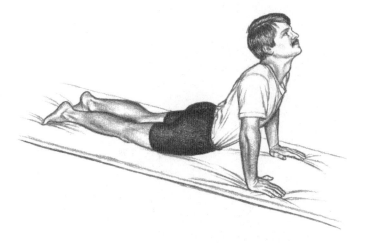

Figure 12. Cobra pose.

VII. LOCUST POSE—*Salabhasana* (30 seconds to 1 minute)

1. Continue to lie facedown and stretch the arms back by your sides, either next to your hips or under the thighs. Face your palms to the ceiling. Bring your feet together and feel the entire back lengthen. Rest your chin gently on the floor.

2. On the inhalation, raise both legs, lengthening them out from your hips. Keep lengthening the entire spine as the legs extend upward and back. Stretch the thighs and keep both legs fully extended and straight. Keep breathing easily, hold for a few breaths, then release the legs down slowly.

3. Repeat the pose 1 to 3 times. Be careful not to hold the breath in this pose. Use the inhalation to lift the legs. Keep lengthening the spine to prevent straining or hyperextending the lower back.

4. Don't force your body to try to achieve a perfect pose. You may wish to raise one leg at a time, lengthening each leg out from the hips, then progressing to raise both legs at once.

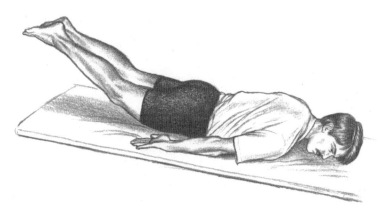

Figure 13. Locust pose.

Benefits: This posture strengthens the lower back, aids in digestion, and benefits the bladder, prostate, uterus, and ovaries.

VIII. SEATED TWISTING POSE—*Marichyasana* (About 1 minute)

1. Sit with the legs extended straight out in front of you. Keep the spine lengthened, the head and neck free.

2. Bend your left knee and keep the sole of the foot on the ground. Bring your heel toward the buttocks just above the inner part of the right knee. The inner side of the your left foot should touch the inner side of the outstretched right thigh. Actively extend your right leg straight out in front of you, lengthening through the back of your leg and heel.

3. Bring your left hand on the floor behind you, and the right arm on the outside of the left knee. If it is difficult to do this, just grasp the knee with your hand. Inhale, lift the rib cage, lengthen your spine vertically upward, and as you exhale, twist from the base of your spine to the left.

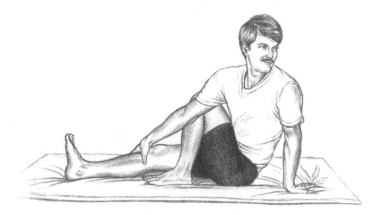

Figure 14. Seated twisting pose.

4. As you twist, keep opening the chest to the left and let your head follow the movement of your spine, following in the direction of the twist. Continue to elongate your spine and open your chest as you breathe. Try not to collapse the front of your body. If you can comfortably keep the spine long in this posture, continue to bring the left hand around the back onto the right thigh. Go only as far as you can without strain.

5. Keep breathing normally and hold the pose for a few breaths. Release slowly, then repeat on the other side. It is especially important to use your breath in this pose and to allow the twist to come from the exhalation. Always twist on a lengthened rather than a compressed spine.

Benefits: This posture increases circulation to the abdominal organs, relieves tightness in the shoulders and upper back, stretches the neck, and stimulates the adrenal glands, liver, and kidneys.

IX. STANDING FORWARD BEND—*Uttanasana* (Up to 1 minute)

1. Stand up and bring your feet together in a parallel position, about hip distance apart. Stand evenly on both feet and lengthen the spine as you lift and open your chest. Keep your head and neck long and free. Look straight ahead and breathe normally.

2. Allow your arms to hang loosely at your sides and keep the shoulders relaxed. Look straight ahead and breathe normally.

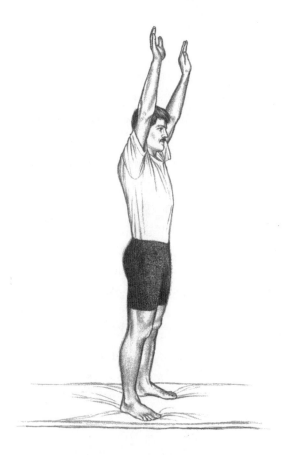

Figure 15.   Standing forward bend.

3. On the inhalation, slowly extend your arms over the head as you lift and expand the chest. On the exhalation, bend the body forward and down, lengthening the entire spine. The arms and head follow in the same line with the spine. Let your knees soften or bend freely and bring your hands to the floor. Keep your elbows and shoulders relaxed and don't lock the knees.

4. Keep breathing easily. Hold the pose for a few breaths. On the inhalation, lift your arms from the upper back as you open the chest forward and up. Come all the way up to a vertical position, arms over your head. Exhale and lower your arms down to the sides.

Benefits: This posture tones the liver, stomach, spleen, kidneys, and spine, and soothes and cools the mind.

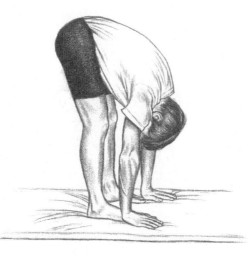

Figure 16.   Standing forward bend.

X. AWARENESS POSE—*Chitasana* (At least 1 minute)

1. Lie down on your back so that both sides of the spine rest evenly on the floor.

2. Lengthen your legs away from the pelvis and let them fall open to the sides. Release your head, neck, shoulders, and hips. Allow the arms to rest loosely next to the body. Face your palms upward.

3. Now let your body be completely relaxed. Close your eyes and rest for at least 1 minute. Allow the breath to be easy and free.

Benefits: This pose invigorates and refreshes both the body and the mind, removes fatigue, and is soothing for the entire system.

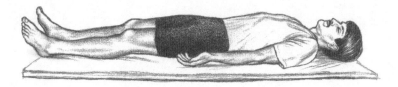

Figure 17. Awareness pose.

BALANCED BREATHING (*Pranayama*)

Time: 5 minutes
Repetitions: 1 set in the morning and 1 set in the evening

Breathing exercises in Ayurveda are a gentle form of balancing the breath—moving from one nostril to the other—a technique called Pranayama. Its purpose is to make the respiratory rhythm more regular, which in turn has a soothing effect on the entire nervous system (that is why we call this a "neurorespiratory" exercise at our Center). A few minutes of balanced breathing, sitting quietly with eyes closed, is very relaxing; many people feel a pleasant lightness in the head afterward and a warm glow inside. Pranayama is the best prelude to meditation, since it effortlessly focuses your attention inward and reduces the scattered thoughts and "noise" that usually fill the mind.

Modern medicine has discovered that brain function is divided between the right and left cerebral hemispheres, each of which contributes its own emphasis. Right-brain activity is intuitive and feeling; left-brain activity is rational and organized. Using the technique of Pranayama, Ayurveda has found a way to "talk" to both hemispheres and bring them into balance. When the breath becomes more balanced, several things happen: you switch your breathing from the right to the left nostril at regular intervals, your mind becomes more clear and alert, and one side of the body is not noticeably weaker than the other.

We recommend 5 minutes of Pranayama morning and evening every day as part of the ideal Ayurvedic daily routine.

A few pointers before you start:

- Any form of straining must be avoided—if you begin to feel dizzy or start to pant, stop for a moment and sit quietly with your eyes closed until you feel normal again. Do not snort in order to clear a clogged nostril. It is not advised to use antihistamines to open your nose before starting. If allergies or a cold have blocked your sinuses, just skip Pranayama until they clear up naturally.
- It is normal for the mucous membranes to contract when you first learn to do this exercise. Just let them relax. Within a few days, they will adjust normally to the new routine.

- Perform Pranayama in a quiet room without radio, music, or TV. Keep your eyes closed. If you feel anxious at any time, stop the exercise for a minute, but do not get up immediately. Sit quietly with your eyes closed until you feel relaxed again. If the uncomfortable sensation persists, lie down for a few minutes until it passes.

- Never hold your breath or count how many seconds you inhale and exhale. These instructions are sometimes seen in yoga books or are given out by yoga teachers. All such practices run contrary to the purpose of this exercise, which is to allow the body to balance the breath itself. Your natural breathing rhythm is right for you.

HOW TO PERFORM BALANCED BREATHING (*Pranayama*)

Find a comfortable chair that allows you to sit upright with your spine straight and both feet on the floor—it is best not to lounge backward while doing Pranayama. Close your eyes, let your mind rest, and place your right hand in the illustrated position—your thumb goes beside your right nostril, your two middle fingers beside your left nostril.

To perform the exercise, gently close one nostril, then the other, as you breathe normally. To keep your arm from getting tired, it helps to tuck your right elbow in close to your ribs, but don't prop it up on your chair or on a table.

The basic rhythm of Pranayama is:

1. Gently close the right nostril with your thumb and slowly exhale through your left nostril. Inhale easily through your left nostril.
2. Close the left nostril with the two middle fingers and exhale out of the right nostril. Inhale easily through the right nostril.

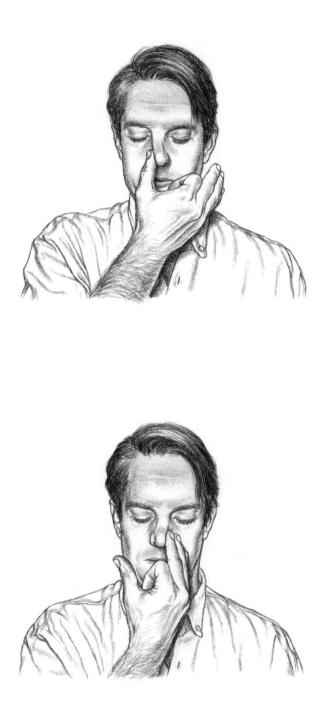

In Pranayama, the hand changes positions with each exhalation of breath.

3. Alternate nostrils for 5 minutes. Then lower your arm and sit back comfortably with eyes closed for 1 or 2 minutes. You can proceed immediately to meditation if that is your next activity.

Note that you *begin each breath on the exhale* and finish on the inhale—this is different from most Western breathing exercises, which begin by taking in a deep breath. In Pranayama, you do not need to take deep breaths. Just let your breathing come naturally but a little slower and deeper than usual. If at any time you feel like breathing through your mouth, go ahead, then return to the exercise as soon as you feel comfortable again. For many people the pattern of breathing changes at times; this is normal and a good sign that you are reaching a more balanced style of respiration.

CHAPTER 14

SEASONAL ROUTINE— BALANCING THE WHOLE YEAR

One of the lessons of the quantum mechanical body is that a person does not stop at the boundary of his skin. His existence continues outward throughout nature. Vata, Pitta, and Kapha are at play everywhere around us, linking our physiologies to the world at large. That is why your body changes with the weather, sensing rain in its bones or growing lazy during the first awakening days of spring. Your doshas are keeping a weather watch for heat, cold, wind, humidity, and all the other variations that the seasons bring.

When a cold, dry wind begins to blow, the Vata inside you responds, because it too is cold, dry, and moving. It senses that something akin to itself has begun to dominate the scene. Each dosha recognizes a particular kind of weather that brings it out, according to the principle of "like speaks to like."

Cold, dry weather, along with wind, accumulates Vata.
Hot weather accumulates Pitta, more so if it is also humid.
Cold, wet weather or snow accumulates Kapha.

The word *accumulate* means that a dosha is increasing in response to surrounding influences; if it increases too much, the accumulation goes on to aggravation, a serious stage of imbalance. The reason a dosha can affect you out of season, as when you get a cold in summer, is that there is a delay, or a spillover effect. It takes time for a dosha to accumulate to the point where it begins to disrupt your body's functioning. The first weeks of autumn may seem perfectly comfortable until you suddenly notice some anxiety or a twinge in your joints, signs of Vata aggravation.

The principle at work here is the same as with a morning hangover: It takes a while for your body to process a mistake and spit it out in the form of a symptom. Vata moves the quickest, so its imbalances tend to show up fastest, followed by Pitta, which might take a month before causing visible trouble, and finally Kapha, which typically remains "stuck" like cold molasses all winter, only to "melt down" and flow in the spring (having a runny nose and sinus problems in April or May indicates that you needed to take better care of Kapha in February).

DOSHAS AND THEIR SEASONS

As with the rhythms of the day, there are master cycles matched to the doshas that run throughout the year. Our bodies automatically flow with these changes as long as we do not interfere. Ayurveda divides the year into three seasons in place of the usual four.

Kapha season falls in spring—mid-March to mid-June.
Pitta season falls in summer and early autumn—mid-June to mid-October.
Vata season bridges late autumn and winter—mid-October to mid-March.

A complete yearly cycle takes us through Kapha, Pitta, and Vata, in that order, mirroring the daily cycle. The calendar season that gets absorbed is autumn, because it is divided between two doshas. Autumn is considered Pitta as long as hot weather prevails and Vata as soon as it turns cold, dry, and windy. People who have a predominance of Vata will walk outside on a crisp October day and feel that the weather is extremely congenial to them—perhaps too much so. The lively, exhilarating quality of fall is only a step away from the fatigue and depression that some people feel at this time of year. The Vata wind seems to fan their inner spark and then blow it out. So one has to be attentive to balancing the whole year, particularly when your body type approaches its vulnerable period.

The three Ayurvedic seasons are only approximate and have to be adjusted according to local conditions. In India, for example, there are six seasons, in keeping with the arrival of the monsoon and other climatic changes that we do not have in the continental United States. On the other hand, many areas of Florida have practically year-round Pitta conditions, giving way to a brief Vata or Kapha winter.

It is not really the calendar but nature itself that tells us when the doshas will be influenced. Any damp, cold, overcast day will cause an increase of Kapha, whether it occurs in fall, winter, or spring. The doshas have the keenest of weather eyes. Even in Florida, they adapt to the minor shifts that prevail in the climate, enabling one to experience a complete cycle of Kapha, Pitta, and Vata during the year.

FOLLOWING A SEASONAL ROUTINE

Traditionally, Ayurveda advises that everyone should follow a seasonal routine (*ritucharya*) to preserve balance as the seasons change. This routine does not involve major alterations in your lifestyle, only a shift of emphasis. You should always maintain your Ayurvedic daily routine—that remains of primary importance—and continue to follow the diet that pacifies your major dosha (or the one specified by a Ayurvedic doctor), with certain variations to blend into the season.

KAPHA SEASON *(Spring and Early Summer)*

Favor a diet that is lighter, drier, and less oily than during other seasons. Heavy dairy products (cheese, yogurt, and ice cream) should be reduced, since they especially tend to aggravate Kapha. Favor warm food and drink. Eat more foods with pungent, bitter, and astringent tastes and fewer with sweet, sour, and salty tastes.

PITTA SEASON *(Midsummer Through Early Autumn)*

Agni is naturally low during hot weather, so you may find that your appetite decreases in summer. Respect this change by not overeating. Favor cool food and drink, but not ice cold. Your body will want more liquids in hot weather, but it is important not to douse the digestive fire by drinking cold liquids after a meal. Favor sweet, bitter, and astringent tastes and reduce sour, salty, and pungent ones.

VATA SEASON *(Late Autumn Through Winter)*

Favor warm food and drink, heavier food, and a more oily diet than you do during the rest of the year. Make sure your food is well cooked and easy to digest, accompanied by plenty of warm liquids (hot water or Vata tea is best). Eat more of the sweet, sour, and salty tastes and less of the bitter, astringent, and pungent. Avoid dry or uncooked foods (especially salads and raw fruits and vegetables). Don't worry if your appetite increases—this is a natural tendency in winter and helps pacify Vata dosha; however, be sure not to eat more than you can comfortably digest.

Two other general points apply:

- Eat fresh produce at all times of year, preferably those that are grown locally.
- Avoid foods that are not locally in season—for example, fewer tomatoes or lettuce in winter, fewer grains in summer, no fruits shipped half-ripened from other locales, and so on.

As you can see, the seasonal routine involves mostly the commonsense adjustments in eating habits that we already follow. But look around a restaurant on a frigid February day and notice how many diners still order chilled salads and ice cream; not knowing any better, almost everyone will be drinking ice water, beer, or cold white wine—all of which are aggravating to Vata during its most prominent season.

In general, the season to be most vigilant about is the one your body type matches—summer for Pittas, winter for Vatas, spring for Kaphas. These are times when you want to be especially faithful to your body-type regimen. Also, at the turn of every season Vata dosha tends to become more vulnerable, so it is good to be careful about Vata when winter turns to spring, spring to summer, and so on, because this is typically when seasonal colds and flu strike.

If you have two doshas prominent in your prakruti, as most people do, you can balance each one as its season comes around. Let's give a practical example. If you are a Vata-Pitta, you would follow a Vata-pacifying diet in late fall and early winter (Vata season) and a Pitta-pacifying diet in summer (Pitta season). The only season left is Kapha, which falls in spring. Here you would blend the Vata diet, which matches your primary dosha, with a Kapha diet, which is naturally suited to the season. To blend two diets means to take half your food from the "favor" column of the Vata diet and half from the "favor" column of the Kapha diet.

Life becomes too complicated if you make an obsession out of changing your diet to suit the weather. The Ayurvedic seasonal routine should be just another way to encourage your body's own natural instincts to emerge.

Epilogue

FLOWERS IN
A QUANTUM FIELD

Most people assume without question that their bodies had a definite beginning and are moving inexorably toward a definite end. Each of us began life as a single cell in the womb and will end as "dust unto dust." However, these are cultural beliefs, not absolute facts. The human body has no definite beginning or end. It is constantly creating itself, again and again, every day. This means that every minute is a kind of genesis and at the same time an ending in which we give up a bit of dust unto dust. If we are creating ourselves all the time, then it is never too late to begin creating the bodies we want instead of the ones we mistakenly assume we are stuck with.

Every breath you take is a creative act. The molecules in the air are random and chaotic. If they happen to enter your body, they magically acquire a purpose and an identity. Could any act be more creative? Consider what happens to a single oxygen atom as you breathe it in. Within a few thousandths of a second it passes through the moist, nearly transparent membranes of the lungs. It immediately attaches itself to the hemoglobin inside one of your red blood cells. In an instant, a remarkable transformation occurs. The blood cell changes color, from the dark blue-black of oxygen-starved hemoglobin to the bright red of oxygen-rich hemoglobin, and a stray atom of air suddenly becomes *you*. It has crossed the invisible boundary dividing the lifeless from the living.

In another sixty seconds the same oxygen atom will make a complete circuit of your body via the bloodstream (the journey takes only fifteen seconds if you are exercising vigorously). In that time, about half of the body's new oxygen will exit the blood to turn into a kidney cell, a biceps muscle, a neuron, or any other tissue. The atom will reside in that tissue anywhere from a few minutes to a year, performing as many functions as you are capable of. An oxygen atom might become part of a happy thought by linking into a neurotransmitter. Or it might instead send a shiver of fear through you by joining a molecule of adrenaline. It could feed a brain cell with glucose or sacrifice itself on the battle line by becoming part of a white cell sent to attack invading bacteria.

This is how the river of life—the river of the body—moves along, with utmost fluidity, intelligence, and creativity. Now that we have surveyed the principles of Ayurveda, it becomes clear that our responsibility to ourselves is also creative. We are placed here in this world to manage a project that is equivalent to building a new universe every day. Creating yourself is not just a full-time job, it is a staggering one. With every single breath, you expose 5 trillion red blood corpuscles to the air. Each corpuscle contains 280 million molecules of hemoglobin. Each molecule of hemoglobin can pick up and transport 8 atoms of oxygen.

If you think of each oxygen atom as a new building block, then with a single breath you are adding 11×10^{21} (or 11,000,000,000,000,000,000,000) new "bricks" that will be delivered to various sites around your body. They will all fit inside you with exact precision, and not a single new brick will disrupt the position of an old one. The old gives way to the new as smoothly and effortlessly as a river runs.

The only reason we are all not perfectly healthy today is that we are constantly taking these infinite new bricks and putting them into the same old slots. Why do we do that? Ultimately it is a matter of awareness, of how we see ourselves. If you look closely at your own life, you will realize that you are sending signals to your body that repeat the same old beliefs, the same old fears and wishes, the same old habits of yesterday and the day before. That is why you are stuck with the same old body.

HANDLING LIFE AS A WHOLE

The new bricks that enter your body do not just fall into place; they are positioned by a bit of inner intelligence that knows how to build your heart, kidneys, skin, enzymes, hormones, DNA, and everything else. This intelligence is literally infinite, and all of it is under our control. Yet, for the most part, we take the boundless creativity of the quantum field and bombard it with narrow beams of attention. Any thought you have is just a beam of focused attention sent out from your quantum self. It takes only a few of these narrow beams, or thoughts, to make life a little longer or a little better. You can add five years to your life, on the average, by deciding to quit smoking. You can add a few more years by losing excess weight or eating good food or taking regular exercise. But these narrow beams of focused attention are limited. They will not make you perfectly healthy. They will not extend your life by two times or ten times, if that is even possible, or improve the quality of life by that much.

It takes breakthrough thinking to do that, as we noted when we began. How can you activate the full potential of your quantum mechanical body? The answer is surprisingly simple. The gigantically complex project of creating yourself can be broken down into just a few processes that come under your control every day:

- *Eating*. Eating is the creative act that selects the raw matter of the world that will be turned into you. To make sure that this process proceeds correctly, you need only to know your body type and follow the diet that matches it. Look back at the section on your body-type diet; let the information sink in by rereading it until you have absorbed the guiding principles. Now eat according to those principles, easily and comfortably.

- *Digestion and assimilation*. Digestion and assimilation are the creative acts that turn the "bricks" of matter into living tissue. Your body's digestive fire, its agni, handles both of these processes, coordinating them perfectly. Look back again at the section on agni, learn how your particular kind functions, and then respect your digestive fire by resetting it regularly.

- *Elimination*. Elimination is the creative act that purifies the body, excreting undigested food and ridding the cells of toxins and other "old bricks." You can improve elimination by being regular in your daily routine and also by taking advantage of Ayurvedic purification therapies. Under the section on agni we talk about purifying herbs; a sattvic diet is also a great help, since it reduces to an absolute minimum the intake of impurities. If you can, incorporate seasonal panchakarma into your annual routine, preferably three times a year or at least once. This is the most powerful therapy for aiding elimination.

- *Breathing*. As the basic rhythm of life that supports all other rhythms, breathing could be called the most creative act we perform with the body. Correct breathing tunes our cells to the rhythms of nature, and the more natural and refined our breathing, the more in tune we become. Many Ayurvedic routines help to bring breathing back into balance—all forms of the three-dosha exercises are good, as well as the gentle Pranayama, or balanced breathing, that you can do for a few minutes every day.

Finally, we can gather all these separate processes under one heading:

Living in tune with your quantum mechanical body. This is the total creative act of life. If you live in tune with your quantum mechanical body, all of your daily activities will proceed as smoothly as the parts—breathing, eating, digestion, assimilation, and elimination. The most important routine to follow here is transcending, the act of getting in touch with the quantum level of yourself. Review the section on meditation and incorporate a few minutes of quieting your mind into your schedule every morning and evening.

According to Ayurveda, this is the way to boost ordinary existence to a higher plane. If we handle a few processes correctly, then the body's own tendency to remain in balance will take care of the rest. At the quantum level, we are all master builders; it is necessary only to follow the guiding intelligence of our nature—our prakruti—and the vast complexity of the body will run as perfectly as the seasons, the tides, and the stars that surround us.

RIPPLES IN THE OCEAN OF CONSCIOUSNESS

At its heart, the "science of life" is a very personal and reassuring kind of knowledge. It returns you to yourself. Now we are ready to send you out on your own to live the knowledge. When you opened this book and read the phrase *perfect health*, you may have been a bit shocked. Every person expects to be sick at some time in his life; to expect otherwise seems almost illegal. Yet the Ayurvedic sages looked at life through different eyes. A famous Vedic verse says, "It is our duty to the rest of mankind to be perfectly healthy, because we are ripples in the ocean of consciousness, and when we are sick, even a little, we disrupt cosmic harmony."

Now you understand the basis for this extraordinary saying. It is not correct to see yourself as an isolated organism in time and space, occupying six cubic feet of volume and lasting seven or eight decades. Rather, you are one cell in the cosmic body, entitled to all the privileges of your cosmic status, including perfect health. Nature made us thinkers so that we could realize this truth. As another Vedic verse declares, "The inner intelligence of the body is the ultimate and supreme genius in nature. It mirrors the wisdom of the cosmos." This genius is inside you, a part of your inner blueprint that cannot be erased.

At the quantum mechanical level, there is no sharp boundary dividing you from the rest of the universe. Each of us is balanced between the infinite and the infinitesimal. The same protons found in the hearts of stars, which have lived at least 5 billion years, take up residence inside us. The neutrinos that streak through the earth in a few millionths of a second are part of us for a brief instant, too. You are a flowing river of atoms and molecules collected from every corner of the cosmos. You are an outcropping of energy whose waves extend to the edges of the unified field. You are a reservoir of intelligence that cannot be exhausted, because nature as a whole is inexhaustible.

Ayurveda has come on the scene at a ripe moment, when "the reenchantment of nature" is taking place at the cutting edge of physics. The idea that the universe is a living, breathing, thinking organism, which would have been ridiculed a generation ago, may prove to be the first principle of a new science. If so, Ayurveda will quickly rise to prominence as the quantum medicine of our time.

For modern man, disease is not a necessity but a choice—nature did not impose a bacterium or virus that causes heart attacks, diabetes, cancer, arthritis, or osteoporosis. These are largely man's dubious creations. But what man has built he can also unbuild. If this book has helped to put your mind on the journey of self-knowledge, you will never again see yourself as trapped by the same old boundaries. If the body, stubborn and solid-looking as it appears, can also undertake this journey, something much greater will be achieved. We will no longer just dream of freedom from the ills that flesh is heir to, we will really become free, clothed in flesh that has become as perfect as our ideals.

Appendix A
SOURCES FOR AYURVEDA

Y ou do not need special supplies or expert advice to balance your doshas and live in accord with Ayurvedic principles. However, there are times in most people's lives when they can use an extra boost to help reestablish optimal health. Specialized foods, spices, and herbs have served an important role in Ayurveda for thousands of years. Many of these traditional products are now available in the West.

Foods: Any wholesome food raised naturally and free of additives is Ayurvedic, but there are also a few specialty foods that make a pleasing addition to the diet:

> *Rose petal jam* is superb for pacifying Pitta and is also considered extremely Sattvic, or pure.
> *Sweetened almond butter* is traditionally considered excellent for vitality and mental alertness.
> If you do not want to take the time to make your own *ghee (clarified butter)*, commercially made varieties are available.

Herbs and food supplements: It is convenient to buy tea bags of specially prepared Vata-, Pitta-, or Kapha-pacifying herb teas, to be alternated with changes in the season. Spice mixtures called *churnas* are also a convenience, since they can be sprinkled over your food at the table to give a Vata-, Pitta-, or Kapha-pacifying effect. More complex, and not duplicable at home, are the traditional rasayanas (herbal food supplements), which often involve dozens of separate preparations and various exotic ingredients.

Aromatic and massage oils: These specially prepared oils are used for abhyanga and aromatherapy and are designed to balance the appropriate dosha.

Miscellaneous: Special raw silk gloves used for *garshana* (dry massage) and silver tongue-scrapers are useful additions to support an ideal daily routine.

A complete line of Ayurvedic products, including Ayurvedically balanced nutritional supplements, can be ordered on the Internet at *MyPotential.com.* Many of these products, foods, or supplements may also be available at your local health food store or Indian grocery.

Visit the Chopra Center for Well Being. Some of the specialized therapies described in this book require supervision by a physician trained in Ayurveda. These include *panchakarma*, the seasonal purification routine, and marma therapy. Courses to enhance wellness and to support individuals facing illness are available year round at the Chopra Center for Well Being in beautiful La Jolla, California. To learn more about the programs and services offered at the Center, call (888) 424-6772 or visit our Web site at www.chopra.com.

Courses in Meditation, Ayurveda, and Mind Body Medicine. We have certified hundreds of instructors throughout the world to offer programs developed at the Chopra Center for Well Being.

For information on any of the following courses, call the Chopra Center at (888) 424-6772 or visit our Web site at www.chopra.com.

Primordial Sound Meditation. Learn an effective mantra meditation technique to quiet your mind, reduce stress, and tap into your reservoir of energy and creativity.

Creating Health. Learn how to apply the principles of Ayurveda to make your daily life happier and healthier.

Magical Beginnings, Enchanted Lives. This course for expectant parents teaches the essential tools for a conscious pregnancy and delivery.

Return to Wholeness. This program guides people facing cancer to their inner place of healing.

MyPotential.com. Visit our new Web site dedicated to helping you reach your highest potential. At *MyPotential.com* you can develop your own program for successful daily living and create a personalized path to fulfilling your dreams and desires.

Appendix B

GLOSSARY

abhyanga—daily oil massage

agni—digestive fire

ama—residual impurities deposited in the body as a result of improper digestion. Also *mental ama*, toxic emotions or negative thoughts as a result of incompletely metabolized emotional experiences

ananda—bliss, synonymous with "pure joy"

asana—a yoga pose

dhatu—one of the body's seven basic constituents, synonymous with "tissue" in Western medicine

dinacharya—the Ayurvedic daily routine

dosha—one of the three basic metabolic principles connecting the mind and body

ghee—clarified butter

guna—any fundamental natural quality (e.g., dry, moist, hot, cold, etc.). Also applied to *sattva, rajas,* and *tamas*—the "three gunas"

Kapha—the dosha responsible for bodily structure

marma—the junction point between consciousness and matter (107 marmas on the skin are accessible through the sense of touch)

ojas—the purest expression of metabolism; the final end product of correct digestion and assimilation of food

panchakarma—purification treatments (literally, "the five actions")

Pitta—the dosha responsible for metabolism

pragya aparadh—the mistake of the intellect (i.e., identifying with the part and losing the whole)

prakruti—nature, referring to one's mind body constitution

Pranayama—Ayurvedic respiratory exercises

rajas—the innate impulse to act

rasa—of the six tastes; also, the first tissue layer (dhatu)

rasayana—Ayurvedic rejuvenative herbal formula

Rishi—a Vedic seer

ritucharya—the Ayurvedic seasonal routine

sattva—purity; the innate impulse to evolve

Surya Namaskar—the "Sun Salute," a twelve-part Ayurvedic physical exercise

tamas—inertia; the innate impulse to remain the same

Vata—the dosha responsible for all movement in the body

Veda—literally "science" or "knowledge." Ayurveda ("the science of life" or "knowledge of lifespan") is an offshoot of Veda.

vipak—the post-digestive effect of food on the body

yoga—Vedic knowledge for attaining union with the domain of pure consciousness. The branch of yoga involving physical exercise is known as *Hatha yoga*.

Bibliography

The following is a selected bibliography that offers insights into some of the ideas expressed in this book.

Chopra, Deepak. *Creating Health.* Boston: Houghton Mifflin Company, 1987.

———. *Quantum Healing: Exploring the Frontiers of Mind/Body Medicine.* New York: Bantam Books, 1989.

———. *Ageless Body, Timeless Mind.* New York: Harmony Books, 1993.

Dash, Bhagwan. *Fundamentals of Ayurvedic Medicine.* Delhi, India: Bansal & Company, 1978.

Frawley, David. *Ayurvedic Healing—A Comprehensive Guide.* Salt Lake City, UT: Passage Press, 1989.

Lad, Vasant. *Ayurveda—The Science of Self-Healing.* Santa Fe, NM: Lotus Press, 1984.

Ranade, Subash. *Natural Healing Through Ayurveda.* Salt Lake City, UT: Passage Press, 1993.

Simon, David. *The Wisdom of Healing.* New York: Harmony Books, 1997.

———. *Vital Energy.* New York: John Wiley & Sons, 2000.

Simon, David, and Deepak Chopra. *The Chopra Center Herbal Guide: Natural Prescriptions for Perfect Health.* New York: Three Rivers Press, 2000.

Svoboda, Robert. *Ayurveda—Life, Health and Longevity.* London: Arkana Penguin Books, 1992.

Index

Abhyanga, 124, 153, 179, 180, 249–53, 378
Abstraction, 75–76, 182
Acne, 155–56, 289
Addiction, 197–211
  curing at home, 208–11
  and doshas, 203–5
  hands–off cure, 200–203
Aftertaste, 286
Aging, 99, 213–25
  quiz on, 225–31
  versus healing, 214–21
  See also Life span
Agni, 254, 293–311, 372
  and ama, 299–300
  body intelligence tips, 309–12
  improving, 301–5
  resetting, 295–99
  throwing off, 299
Air, 76
Alcohol, 197, 200, 205, 210, 255
Allen, Betsy, 190
Alochaka Pitta, 83–84
Aloe vera, 223
Ama, 118, 129, 145, 152, 299–300, 314
  See also Mental ama
Amoeba, 23
Angina, 171–72, 173, 174
Anthropic principle, 16
Apana Vata, 81–82
Aromatherapy, 187–91, 210, 378
Arteries, 8, 14, 215–16
Assimilation, 372
Astringency, 257–58, 286, 292–93
Atom, 168
Attention, 175–78
Attitude, 21
Avalambaka Kapha, 85
Awareness, 11, 13, 28, 147–49, 217
Awareness pose, 358
Aygen, M.M., 165
Ayurveda:
  balance in, 25–26, 92
  definition of, 11
  desire to lift all aspects of life, 47

  disease process in, 117–19
  natural impulses in, 238–39
  sources for, 377–79
  See also Doshas

Back pain, 155
Balance:
  in Ayurveda, 25–26
  and body type, 38
  in doshas, 68–69, 92–93, 120–33
  as flexible, 74–75
  of gunas, 72
  perfect, 91
  restoring, 109–34
Balanced breathing, 318, 325, 358–62
Basti, 154
Beans, 268, 275, 282
Bedtime, 247, 255–56
Bhodaka Kapha, 85
Bhrajaka Pitta, 84
Biochavan, 224
Biochemical individuality, 32
Biological age, 218–20
BITS (body intelligence tips), 309–12
Bitter taste, 258, 286, 290–91
Bliss, 181–85, 306
Blubber, 73
Body:
  characteristics of types, 46–47
  as intelligent, 137, 146, 236, 371, 374
  mind body connection, 26, 36, 117, 139, 140, 178
  respecting type, 88–90
  as "river," 18–19, 369–70, 374
  thermostat, 111–12
  See also Quantum mechanical human body
Bowel movements, 248
Brahmi Rasayana, 224
Brain, 25, 111
Breakthrough thinking, 9
Breathing, 372–73
  See also Balanced breathing

Index

Cabbage, 285–86
Canker sore, 65
Cardiovascular disease, 227
Cells, 23–24, 146, 178, 215–18
Chakras, 172–73
Charaka, 317
Chavanprash, 224
Choices, 237–41
Cholesterol, 164–65
Chronological age, 218–19
Churnas, 266, 272, 378
Cobra pose, 352–53
Compassion, 210
Complementarity, 222
Conventional medicine, 32, 116
Cooper, M.J., 165
Coronary arteries, 8, 14
Cures, 28–29

Daily routine, 120, 243–56
Dairy, 268, 274, 282
Death, 10
De Luca, Cheryl, 155–56
Depression, 140, 160–61
Desire, 235–40
DHEA (dehydroepiandrosterone), 220
Diet, 121, 257–315, 372
    balanced, 257–58
    body intelligence tips, 309–12
    body-type, 259–62
    and canker sores, 65–66
    fresh food, 314
    and imbalances, 66, 120
    Kapha-pacifying, 131, 276–83, 368
    and natural adaptation, 73
    non-ojas, 313–14
    Pitta-pacifying, 126–27, 270–76, 368
    pleasing additions to, 377
    sattvic, 306–9
    Vata-pacifying, 123, 262–69, 367–68
Digestion. See Agni
Dinacharya. See Daily routine
Dinner, 247, 254–55
Disease. See Sickness and disease
DNA, 15, 24, 73, 145, 213–18
Doshas, 36–38
    and addiction, 203–5
    aggravating, 92–93
    balancing, 68–69, 92–93, 120–21, 188
    as blueprint from nature, 87–108

and diet, 258–59
and digestion, 294–95
gunas, 69–75
imbalances, 65, 66, 94–95, 98–108
learning to "see," 63–68
pacifying, 115
and seasons, 364–68
seats of, 66, 67
subdoshas, 77–86
types, 45, 57–61
See also Kapha; Pitta; Vata
Drug addiction, 197–203, 205, 210
Dry (guna), 71
Dry massage. See Garshana

Earth, 76
Eating. See Diet
Elecampane, 223
Elements. See Five elements
Elimination, 372
Enema. See Basti
Energy, 75
Environment, 22
Eskimos, 73
Exercise, 120, 132, 317–62
    balanced breathing, 318, 325, 358–62
    body-type, 320–24
    myth of no pain, no gain, 319–20
    precautions, 324–25
    Sun Salute, 318, 325
    yoga, 318, 325, 339–58

Fatigue, 146
Fire, 76
Five elements, 75–77
Five senses. See Senses
"Flow" periods, 185
Food. See Diet; specific foods
Frazier, Daniel, 155
Free radicals, 225
Freud, Sigmund, 206
Fruits, 267, 273–74, 281

Garshana, 132, 133–34, 378
Genetics, 46
Ghee, 272, 304, 377
Ginger, 264, 278, 301–3
Glaser, Jay, 220

Goleman, Daniel, 17
Gotu kola, 223, 224, 264
Grains, 267, 274, 282
Grief, 99–100
Growth, 25–26
Gunas, 69–75, 77, 130, 238, 257, 260

Habits, 230
Happiness, 140, 228
Headaches, 160–61, 163
Head to knee pose, 346–48
Healing:
  sounds, 167–68, 174–75
  techniques, 151–95
  versus aging, 214–21
  visualization, 175–78
  See also specific techniques
Heart, 78
Heart attack, 139–40, 141
Heart disease, 8, 14, 15, 73, 227
Heavy (guna), 72
Helicobacter pylori, 96
Heraclitus, 18
Herbs, 221–25, 269, 276, 283, 285, 305,
  377–78
Holmes, Ann, 78–80
Honey, 223, 279
Host resistance/defenses, 8, 98
Hot (guna), 72
Hunger, 127, 297, 311
Hypertension, 163–64, 165, 288–89
Hypnosis, 140–41
Hypothalamus, 25, 111, 112, 188, 235

Immune system, 142
Incurable illness, 28–29
Indian food, 223
Indians, 73
Insomnia, 110
Instinct, 120–21
Intelligence, 15–16, 18, 178, 182, 229
  and aging, 215, 218
  and balance, 112
  of body, 137, 146, 236, 371, 374
Intention, 175–78

James, William, 21
Job satisfaction, 140, 227
Joy. *See* Bliss

Kapha, 44
  balancing, 129–33, 189
  body-type quiz, 42–44
  characteristics of, 53–56
  and daily routine, 243–44
  diet, 131, 258–61, 276–83, 287–90,
    368
  digestion, 294, 296
  exercise for, 132, 317, 320, 321,
    323–24
  and five elements, 76–77
  and five senses, 187
  flavor of joy, 183
  fundamental qualities, 69, 71
  imbalance, 74, 93, 104–8
  physical disorders, 94
  positive psychological traits, 91
  pure body type, 57
  and seasons, 364–68
  subdoshas, 84–86
Kapha-Pitta, 45, 59–60
Kapha-Vata, 45, 60–61
Kledaka Kapha, 84
Knowledge, 217–18

Lassi, 265–66, 309
Laxative treatment. *See* Virechana
Leftovers, 314
Leukemia, 141–49
Life span, 22–24, 217, 220
  herbs for longevity, 221–25
Liver, 222
Locust pose, 353–54
Longevity. *See* Life span
Lunch, 247, 254, 314

Mantras, 161, 173
Marma therapy, 178–86
  clinical, 179–80
  at home, 180–81
Maslow, Abraham, 184–85
Massage:
  abhyanga, 124, 153, 179, 180, 249–53,
    378
  garshana, 132, 133–34, 378
Master cycles, 243–44, 364
Matter, 75, 138
Meat, 268, 275, 282
Meditation, 122–23, 126, 130, 157–67, 254
  and addiction, 201–3, 209

Meditation (*continued*)
  and aging, 219–21, 231
  learning how, 167
  as medicine, 163–67
  for mind healing itself, 160–63
Melanoma, 26–28
Memory. *See* Smriti
Meningococcus bacteria, 7–8
Menstruation, 78–80
Mental ama, 157, 239–40, 312
Metabolic principles, 63
Metabolism, 37
Mexico, 284
Milk, 284, 308
Mills, Joan, 248
Mind body connection, 26, 36, 117,
  139, 140, 178
Minerals, 236
Moderation, 125, 311
Movement, 37
Multiple personality disorder,
  16–18
Music therapy, 191–95, 209

Nasya (nasal treatment), 154
Natural adaptation, 73
Nature:
  accessing bliss of, 181–82
  as blueprint, 87–108
  healing sounds in, 167–68
  impulse to evolve, 235–42
  living in tune with, 235, 244
  reenchantment of, 21–25
  through five senses, 182–83
Neal, Patsy, 184
Needs, 235–36
Neuromuscular integration. *See*
  Yoga
Nutrition, 257
Nuts, 264, 268, 275, 283

Oil massage. *See* Abhyanga
Oils, 268, 275, 283
Ojas, 306, 309–10, 312–14
Oleation. *See* Snehana
Olfactory cells, 188
Omega-3 fats, 73
Orme-Johnson, David, 165, 167
Ornish, Dean, 14, 15
Oxygen, 370

Pachaka Pitta, 82–83
Pain, 79, 96
Panchakarma, 79, 145–46, 152–56
  and aging, 230–31
  case studies, 154–56
  steps of, 153–54
  today, 156
Peak experiences, 184–85
Peptic ulcers, 96–97
Perfect health, 29, 240, 371, 374
  and body type, 33–35
  choosing, 10
  definition of, 7–10
  as possibility, 25, 143
PET (positron-emission tomography), 138
Phantom pain, 96
Physical function, 228
Pineal gland, 74
Pitta, 44
  balancing, 125–29, 189
  body-type quiz, 40–42
  characteristics of, 50–53
  and daily routine, 243–44
  diet, 126–27, 258–60, 270–76, 288–90,
    368
  digestion, 294, 296
  exercise for, 317, 320, 322–23
  and five elements, 76
  and five senses, 187
  flavor of joy, 183
  fundamental qualities, 69, 70–71
  imbalance, 93, 96–97, 102–4
  physical disorders, 94
  positive psychological traits, 91
  pure body type, 57
  and seasons, 364–68
  subdoshas, 82–84
Pitta-Kapha, 45, 59
Pitta-Vata, 45, 58–59
Plaque, 216
Plow pose, 350–52
Prakruti, 33, 35, 88, 90–91, 112, 114
Prana Vata, 77, 80–81
Pranayama. *See* Balanced breathing
Prigogine, Ilya, 21
Primordial sound, 171
Primordial Sound Meditation, 157, 167
Psycho-physiological constitutional
  type, 35
Pulse, 65
Pungency, 257, 258, 286, 291–92
Pure joy, 182

Quality at the source, 10
Quantum, definition of, 12, 168
Quantum mechanical human body,
    12–18, 27–28, 372
    and aging, 213–31
    channels of healing, 151–95
    impulse to evolve, 235–42
    living in tune with, 373
    quantum medicine for, 137–49
Quantum physics, 169
Quantum principle, 13
Quantum reality, 168–70

Rajas, 238–39
Ranjaka Pitta, 83
Rasas. *See* Tastes
Rasayanas, 115, 221–25, 230
Red chilies, 284
Regularity, 122
Rest, 122, 126
Rice, Gerald, 141–49
Rising time, 246, 248–50
Ritucharya. *See* Seasonal routine

SAD (seasonal affective disorder), 74
Sadhaka Pitta, 83
Saffron, 223
Salt, 258, 272, 285, 288–89
Samana Vata, 81
Samhita, 217
Satisfaction, 200–201
Sattva, 238–39, 240–42
Sattvic diet, 306–9, 313
Schmitt, Andreas, 26–28
Seasonal routine, 120, 363–68
Seated twisting pose, 354–55
Seat-firming pose, 345, 346
Seeds, 268, 275, 283
Self-actualized individuals, 184
Self-image, 114
Senses, 144, 182–83, 187
Shleshaka Kapha, 86
Shoulder stand, 348–50
Sickness and disease:
    and body type, 33–34
    cause of, 7–8
    differences among diseases, 32
    emotional resistance to, 8–9
    individualizing, 34–35
    and mind body connection, 26

prevention, 34, 120
    quantum medicine, 139–49
    self-health rating, 229
    six stages of, 116–19
    spontaneous remissions, 28–29
    subtle sources of, 95–98
Silence, 158, 159, 162
Sleep, 122, 245
Smell, 188–89
Smoking, 197, 200, 206–8, 228
Smriti, 198, 216
Snehana, 153
Sound, 77, 167–68, 171–75
Sour taste, 258, 286, 289–90
Space, 76, 77
Spices, 269, 276, 283, 285, 305, 377–78
Spicy foods, 264, 278, 291–92
Spontaneous remissions, 28–29
Standing forward bend, 356–57
Stimulation, 129
Stress, 114, 115, 146, 201, 210
Stress hormones, 157
Structure, 37
Sun Salute, 318, 325, 326–39
Superconductivity, 186
Superfluidity, 185–86
Sweat treatments. *See* Swedana
Swedana, 154
Sweetness, 258, 268, 275, 283, 285–88
Swimming, 323

Tamas, 238–39
Tarpaka Kapha, 85–86
Tastes, 188, 257–58, 260, 283–93
Tea, 263–64, 271, 301, 377–78
Thomas, Bobby, 88–90
Thoughts, 138
Tongue, 248–49
Toxic residues. *See* Panchakarma

Udana Vata, 81
Understanding, 210
Unified field, 169–70, 171

Varicella virus, 8
Vata, 37–38, 44, 68–69, 325
    and addiction, 204–5
    aggravation, 99, 114–15, 204
    balancing, 121–25, 189

Vata (*continued*)
  body-type quiz, 38–40
  case study, 88–90
  characteristics of, 47–50
  and daily routine, 243–44
  diet, 123, 258–60, 262–69, 290–91,
    367–68
  digestion, 294, 296
  exercise for, 317, 320, 321–22
  and five elements, 76
  and five senses, 187
  flavor of joy, 183
  fundamental qualities, 69, 70
  imbalance, 46, 66, 79, 93, 95–96,
    98–102, 204
  physical disorders, 94
  positive psychological traits, 91
  pure body type, 57
  and seasons, 364–68
  subdoshas, 77, 80–82
Vata-Kapha, 45, 60
Vata-Pitta, 45, 58, 367
Vata-Pitta-Kapha, 45–46

Vegetables, 266, 273, 280–81
Vikruti, 113–15
Violence, 240
Vipak. *See* Aftertaste
Virechana, 127–28, 153
Virtual energy, 13
Vitamins, 236
Vyana Vata, 82

Walking, 317, 323
Wallace, Robert Keith, 201, 219,
  220
Water, 76
Weight, 91–92, 230, 312

Yoga, 179, 323, 325, 339–58
  See also specific poses
Yogurt, 66

Zero defects, 9–10